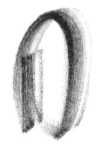

APPLE CIDER VINEGAR DRINKS

for Health

100 Teas, Seltzers, Smoothies,

Incr   ion

Ease   iant

$15.99

BRITT BRANDON, CFNS, CPT

Adams Media
New York London Toronto Sydney New Delhi

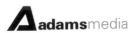

Adams Media
An Imprint of Simon & Schuster, Inc.
57 Littlefield Street
Avon, Massachusetts 02322

First Adams Media trade paperback edition June 2018

ADAMS MEDIA and colophon are trademarks of Simon & Schuster.

For information about special discounts for bulk purchases, please contact Simon & Schuster Special Sales at 1-866-506-1949 or business@simonandschuster.com.

The Simon & Schuster Speakers Bureau can bring authors to your live event. For more information or to book an event contact the Simon & Schuster Speakers Bureau at 1-866-248-3049 or visit our website at www.simonspeakers.com.

Interior design by Heather McKiel
Photographs by James Stefiuk

Manufactured in the United States of America

10 9 8 7 6 5 4 3 2 1

Library of Congress Cataloging-in-Publication Data
Brandon, Britt, author.
Apple cider vinegar drinks for health / Britt Brandon, CFNS, CPT.
Avon, Massachusetts: Adams Media, 2018.
Series: For health.
Includes index.
LCCN 2018003625 (print) | LCCN 2018005917 (ebook) | ISBN 9781507207567 (pb) | ISBN 9781507207574 (ebook)
LCSH: Cider vinegar--Health aspects. | Cider vinegar--Therapeutic use. | BISAC: COOKING / Health & Healing / General. | HEALTH & FITNESS / Alternative Therapies. | HEALTH & FITNESS / Healing.
LCC RM666.V55 (ebook) | LCC RM666.V55 B75 2018 (print) | DDC 615.3/23642--dc23
LC record available at https://lccn.loc.gov/2018003625

ISBN 978-1-5072-0756-7
ISBN 978-1-5072-0757-4 (ebook)

Contents

Introduction

Cultures around the globe have used apple cider vinegar (also known as ACV) for centuries in their treatment of illnesses. Today, millions of people use this beneficial product to treat conditions such as indigestion, anxiety, sinus issues, colds and flus, toxicity, brain "fog," insomnia, and even chronic conditions that can result in debilitating health issues. A simple tablespoon of ACV, consumed daily, can give you immeasurable health benefits, such as weight loss, better immunity, improved digestion, increased energy, and so much more!

This book will share with you how easy it can be to incorporate a daily dose of ACV into your life. With delicious combinations of nutrient-dense fruits and vegetables, protein-packed yogurts, aromatic spices, tasty teas, fizzy kombuchas, and surprise additions that add an abundance of essential nutrients, you can sip your way to better health. To make things even easier, this book is separated into chapters that address specific areas of health, so you can quickly find the right recipes to meet your particular health needs.

Because of ACV's notoriously bitter taste, many people choose to combine it with another liquid, such as water. But you don't have to limit yourself to water when there is a whole cornucopia of healthy and delicious ingredients to add to ACV to make superpowered nutritional drinks. With this book, anyone can create delicious and nutritious elixirs that combine the benefits of ACV with a wide variety of nutrients and potent antioxidants to improve almost every area of life!

With these delicious ACV tonics, you can ensure your body's proper functioning and provide your body's cells, organs, and systems with protective enzymes and nutrients. So, let's get ready to start your journey to better health with a time-tested ingredient that can help you transform your body and mind!

Chapter 1

ALL ABOUT APPLE CIDER VINEGAR

Many people are turning to all-natural healing approaches, and with its tried-and-true results, apple cider vinegar (ACV) has become a staple in the health world. ACV helps to detoxify the body and brain; improve the circulatory, respiratory, and immune systems; and maintain proper digestive functioning. It has been shown to improve blood sugar levels, protect your heart health, and help you lose weight. However, there is one downside to apple cider vinegar: its tart, sour taste. Fortunately, ACV can be added to delicious and nutritious culinary creations that make its daily consumption something to look forward to! As you'll see in the recipes in this book, ACV blends well with sweet fruits and berries, deep greens, creamy yogurts, nuts, and natural juices, so you can reap the many health benefits of ACV without the dreaded vinegar taste.

What Is Apple Cider Vinegar?

Apple cider vinegar (ACV) is apple cider that has been fermented using yeast. The natural sugars within the fruit are broken down by the yeast and bacteria and turned into alcohol—this is the fermentation process. The alcohol then undergoes a second fermentation process, and voilà! Vinegar. While a wide variety of carbohydrates can be used to create vinegar, apples are the only source that provides the unique taste and health benefits of ACV.

Apple cider vinegar has been a kitchen staple for decades, but few people are aware of its powerful uses beyond a splash on a salad or a dash in a dish. The organic, unfiltered variety of ACV is very different from the regular apple cider vinegar that is on almost every grocery store shelf. The difference between the organic, unfiltered variety and the heavily processed version is in how the vinegars are produced. Organic apple cider vinegar is more nutritious and boasts more health benefits. You can visually tell the difference between organic and non-organic apple cider vinegar by looking at them. Organic ACV has a slightly cloudy appearance, with sediment in the bottom of the bottle. Non-organic ACV is clear, without any visible particles. This is because the non-organic variety has undergone pasteurization—a process in which a substance is heated and distilled. The pasteurization process kills many of the naturally occurring bacteria, nutrients, and enzymes in the apple cider vinegar—commonly referred to as "the mother"—and all the health-boosting properties they contain.

"The Mother" in Apple Cider Vinegar

Apple cider vinegar contains an all-powerful "mother"—the cobweb- or sediment-like substance that can be seen floating in unfiltered varieties of ACV. "The mother" contains the concentrated bacteria and enzymes that give ACV the antifungal, antiviral, and antibacterial healing powers for which it has become so famous. While some people may be put off by the sediment in their ACV bottles, this element is the result of the specific processing that retains the nutrients and enzymes of the apples throughout the fermentation process, and thereby provides ACV's unique healing powers.

The Beneficial Nutrients of ACV

Apples are packed with vitamins and minerals that give ACV its myriad health benefits. The key is to buy raw, unfiltered apple cider vinegar. Because of the careful process that is used to create this variety of ACV, the essential nutrients that are so sought after remain intact and unadulterated. Here are the vitamins present and their health benefits:

- Vitamin A: for eye health; also a powerful antioxidant
- Vitamin B_1: for nervous system functioning, digestive health, and muscle health
- Vitamin B_2: for healthy skin, hair, and nails; also aids in breakdown of proteins, carbohydrates, and fats
- Vitamin B_6: for alleviating skin conditions and nerve damage; also assists in utilization of proteins, carbohydrates, and fats
- Vitamin B_{12}: for red blood cell formation and proper nerve cell functioning
- Vitamin C: for immune system functioning; also a powerful antioxidant
- Vitamin E: for skin and nerve health; also a powerful antioxidant

There are also a number of minerals found in raw, unfiltered ACV:

- Calcium: for bone health
- Chromium: for regulating blood glucose
- Copper: for nerve functioning, bone maintenance, and proper utilization of glucose
- Iron: for transport of oxygen and blood health
- Magnesium: for synthesis of proteins and cellular energy production
- Manganese: for formation and maintenance of bone, as well as carbohydrate metabolism
- Phosphorous: for proper cell functioning and strong bones
- Potassium: for muscle contraction, nerve impulses, and energy production
- Selenium: for fat metabolism; also has antioxidant properties
- Sodium: for maintaining proper fluid balance
- Zinc: for promoting healing

Apples (and apple cider vinegar) also contain pectin, which has been shown to aid in digestion. That's how ACV is able to act as a cleansing agent and assist the colon in ridding the body of toxins and waste that have built up over time. The pectin in ACV forms a gel-like substance that attaches to debris in the digestive system and helps carry it away naturally.

Integrating ACV Into Your Daily Life

The simple addition of ACV into your daily routine will give you vast and plentiful health benefits. From glowing skin and better focus to improved digestion and regulated hormonal production, the results of ingesting ACV can be life altering. Apple cider vinegar has a lot of potential uses, from beauty products to home cleaning applications, but in terms of ingesting it for health, there are a few things to be aware of. First of all, this is a vinegar, so it is highly acidic and sour tasting. It is not something you would want to (or should) drink straight. Apple cider vinegar should always be diluted or mixed into a drink like the ones in this book. There is no set dosage of apple cider vinegar, but most people take anywhere from a teaspoon to a tablespoon (diluted in some way) up to three times a day.

SOME CAVEATS

Apple cider vinegar is a natural product and is safe for your consumption. However, there are two groups of people who should consult with their doctors before consuming ACV on a regular basis. While ACV does contain some calcium, women with osteoporosis should speak with their doctors, as regular use of ACV can reduce bone density. People with diabetes should also check with their doctors before starting an ACV program, as ACV can alter insulin levels in some people.

Tips for Purchasing and Storing ACV

Because apple cider vinegar has grown in popularity in just the past few years, the product can be found in almost every health store, grocery store, and drugstore. While these readily available versions of ACV may seem convenient and enticing, many of these are the filtered, non-organic versions that provide absolutely no benefit in terms of health. When purchasing the ACV that promotes health, healing, and overall well-being, make sure the product states that the vinegar is unfiltered, unpasteurized, and organic, while also promoting the presence of "the mother."

All bottles of apple cider vinegar should have an expiration date printed on them. ACV is typically fine for up to five years (even after opening it). The expiration date on the bottle mostly refers to the date when the flavor and quality of the vinegar will begin to falter. You don't have to follow any special procedures after you break the seal on your bottle of ACV. Because of the high acidity of the vinegar, there is no chance of it "going bad" or developing mold as long as you use it by the date marked. You also don't need to refrigerate your opened bottle of apple cider vinegar. However, to preserve the flavor you should keep the bottle tightly capped and in a cool, dry, and preferably dark place, like a pantry or cellar. ACV can become cloudy over time, but it is still safe to consume if this happens.

Chapter 2

RECIPES FOR WEIGHT LOSS

A growing percentage of the population is searching for ways to achieve effective, long-lasting weight loss. With the availability of countless programs, pills, products, and potions promising weight loss success, many consumers fall prey to marketing ploys for products that fail to deliver. However, apple cider vinegar's nutrients and enzymes work synergistically to improve the functioning of the body's cells, organs, and systems, and the physical results are often seen in significant, sustainable, natural weight loss. With an improved digestive system that absorbs key nutrients and expels waste properly, regulated hormones that improve energy and control satiety, and a metabolism that helps burn fat and retain muscle, your body is better able to maintain a healthy weight. Apple cider vinegar is one of the healthiest ingredients you can add to your diet for successful weight loss. With sweet fruits like berries and citrus, and deep greens that add fiber and antioxidants, the apple cider vinegar concoctions in this chapter will help you enjoy your daily dose of ACV and shed pounds at the same time.

DARK CHOCOLATE CHERRY

Serves 2
INGREDIENTS

1 tablespoon apple cider vinegar
2 cups pitted cherries
1 ounce dark chocolate
2 cups unsweetened vanilla almond
  milk
1 cup ice

1 Combine all the ingredients in a large blender.
2 Blend the ingredients on high until thoroughly combined and frothy.
3 Consume immediately or store tightly sealed and unrefrigerated up to 4 hours.

KEY INGREDIENT: Dark Chocolate

Most people consider chocolate to be the treat that derails diets and contributes to caloric overload. While many commercial milk-chocolate products contain high amounts of sugar and additives that can be detrimental to health, dark chocolate has more health benefits than you might think. With plentiful potent antioxidants that serve to protect cells against free radical damage, dark chocolate (in small amounts) has been shown to curb cravings for sweets. When combined with the rich flavors of vibrant fruits and vegetables, protein-rich additions, and health-improving apple cider vinegar, the benefits to the brain and body are immeasurable! A small serving of dark chocolate can actually assist in a weight loss program by satisfying the sweet tooth, increasing the probability of opting for a nutritious snack rather than an unhealthy alternative, and protecting cells and promoting energy levels naturally.

Per Serving
Calories: 220 | Fat: 10 g | Protein: 4 g | Sodium: 190 mg
Fiber: 6 g | Carbohydrates: 33 g | Sugar: 23 g

TANGY TARRAGON WATERMELON

Serves 2
INGREDIENTS

1 tablespoon apple cider vinegar
4 cups watermelon chunks
2 tablespoons chopped fresh tarragon
1 teaspoon honey
2 cups purified water (pH-balanced)

1 Combine all the ingredients in a large blender.
2 Blend the ingredients on high until thoroughly combined and frothy.
3 Consume immediately or store tightly sealed and unrefrigerated up to 4 hours.

KEY INGREDIENT: Watermelon

Packed with water that drips from the smiling mouths of children every summer, this delicious melon also provides a number of nutrients, from micronutrients, like vitamins and minerals, to macronutrients, like carbohydrates, that help stave off hunger and satisfy cravings. When concerned with weight loss, any snack, smoothie, or meal that can have watermelon added is an automatic weight loss winner! The fiber helps keep you feeling full longer, the sweetness satisfies your sweet tooth, the low caloric content makes for a no-worry addition, and the flavor can be combined with other fruits, vegetables, and an assortment of aromatic herbs. With the benefits of this beautiful fruit helping to improve the taste of your daily diet and maximize your weight loss, you'll love this delicious and nutritious combination of wonderful watermelon and astounding apple cider vinegar.

Per Serving
Calories: 100 | Fat: 0.5 g | Protein: 2 g | Sodium: 5 mg
Fiber: 1 g | Carbohydrates: 26 g | Sugar: 22 g

SWEET GREEN BANANA

Serves 2

INGREDIENTS

1 tablespoon apple cider vinegar
2 cups spinach leaves
1 medium banana, peeled
2 cups organic apple juice
1 cup ice

1 Combine all the ingredients in a large blender.

2 Blend the ingredients on high until thoroughly combined and frothy.

3 Consume immediately or store tightly sealed and unrefrigerated up to 4 hours.

KEY INGREDIENT: Spinach

Full of fiber and rich in valuable nutrients, including iron and vitamins A, C, E, and K, this leafy green vegetable is an amazing addition to any weight loss diet. With its combination of calcium, iron, and zinc all helping the body to absorb and utilize vitamins and minerals as needed for optimal metabolism, spinach is the healthy core of this apple cider vinegar drink. By getting the daily requirement of important vitamins, minerals, and antioxidants *while* filling up on fiber, your body's cells and systems get what they need to function properly. Combine that with extra energy, stamina, and mental clarity, and your body is primed for weight loss. With filling fiber, you also reap the benefits of feeling satisfied longer after a spinach-packed snack or meal, making this low-calorie, nutrient-rich addition a weight loss win-win!

Per Serving
Calories: 180 | Fat: 0.5 g | Protein: 2 g | Sodium: 50 mg
Fiber: 2 g | Carbohydrates: 45 g | Sugar: 37 g

COOL CUCUMBER MELON

Serves 2

INGREDIENTS

1 tablespoon apple cider vinegar
2 medium cucumbers, peeled and chopped
2 cups chopped honeydew melon
1 tablespoon honey
2 cups purified water (pH-balanced)

1 Combine all the ingredients in a large blender.

2 Blend the ingredients on high until thoroughly combined and frothy.

3 Consume immediately or store tightly sealed and unrefrigerated up to 4 hours.

KEY INGREDIENT: Honey

Many people who are focused on losing weight are conscious of the amount of sugar that they consume throughout the day. While the amount of sugar you ingest does play a major role in weight gain and weight loss, it is always important to consider the source of that sugar. While sugar packets, artificial sweeteners, and high-fructose corn syrup products contribute to countless health conditions, honey is a sweet superfood that rarely gets the attention it deserves. Wonderful for sweetening drinks, smoothies, snacks, and delectable dishes, honey not only provides a taste of sweetness, but it does so without spiking blood sugar or contributing to hormonal fluctuations. The sweetness of honey also balances beautifully with the tartness of apple cider vinegar in this delicious recipe.

Per Serving
Calories: 120 | Fat: 1 g | Protein: 2 g | Sodium: 35 mg
Fiber: 3 g | Carbohydrates: 28 g | Sugar: 25 g

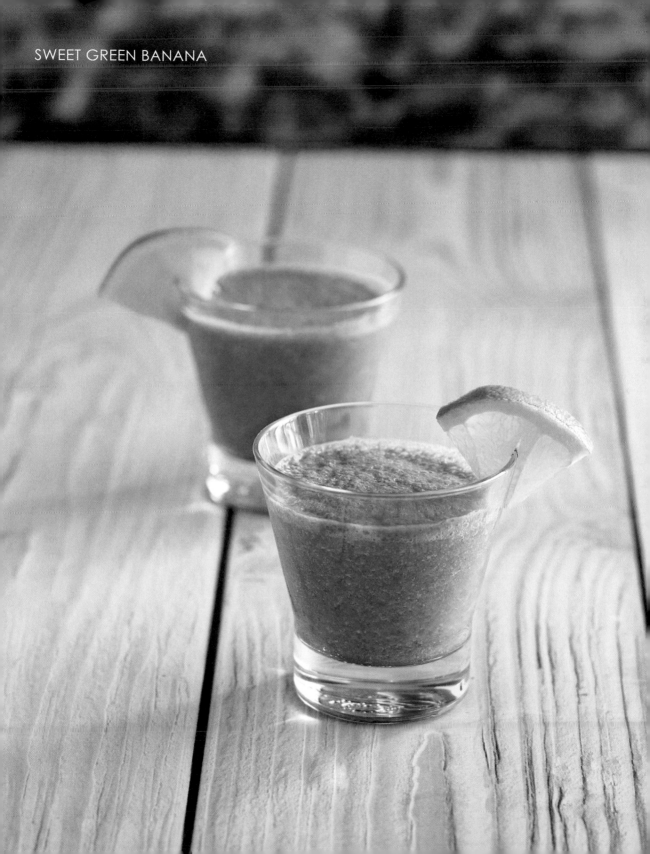

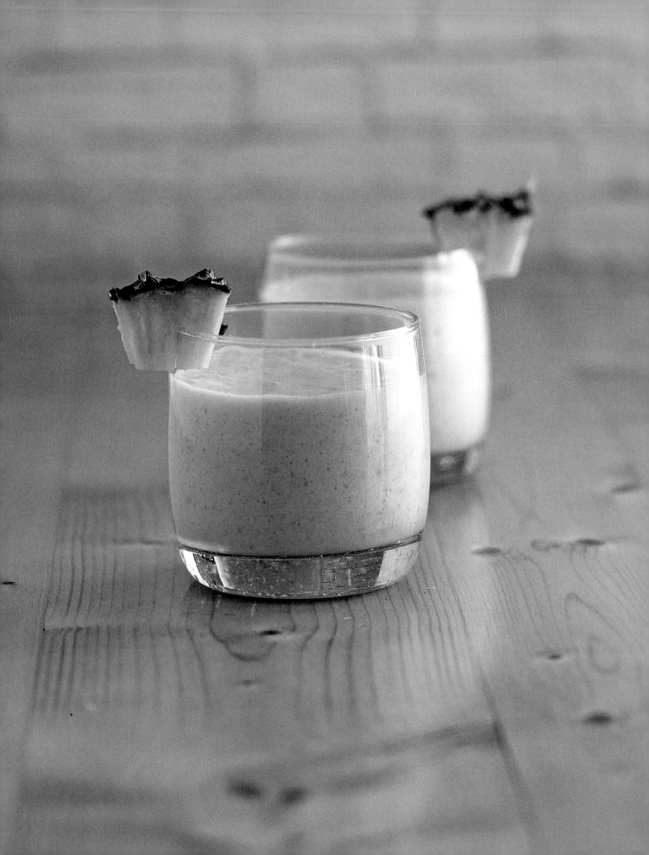

TROPICAL TREAT

Serves 2

INGREDIENTS

1 tablespoon apple cider vinegar
2 medium bananas, peeled and
   frozen
1 cup chopped pineapple
1 cup ice
2 cups low-fat coconut milk

---

1 Combine all the ingredients in
   a large blender.

2 Blend the ingredients on high
   until thoroughly combined and
   frothy.

3 Consume immediately or store
   tightly sealed and refrigerated
   up to 4 hours.

KEY INGREDIENT: Banana

Bananas were long thought to be an enemy in the weight loss battle, but this is simply not true. Bananas contain fiber and resistant starch (starch that is not completely digested), and while they may be higher in carbohydrates than other fruits, bananas are a low glycemic index food, so they do not adversely affect your blood sugar. It is the fiber in bananas that is the true weight loss and digestive helper here though. Fiber plays an important role in weight loss because it helps slow down the digestive process, helping you feel fuller for longer and keeping your blood sugar balanced. If you're feeling full you are less likely to go searching for unhealthy foods to fill the void, and if your blood sugar is balanced your body will burn excess fat for energy. Additionally, bananas are low-energy-density food, meaning that they give you more food with less calories than others foods, because they have extra bulk from things like water and fiber. Packed with digestive-friendly fiber, this sweet addition can infuse your apple cider vinegar drinks with a tropical-island feel. Since weight loss success depends on energy production, balanced blood sugar, and the ability to not feel hungry or deprived, a banana's nutrients and fiber make winning a weight loss battle simple and sweet.

Per Serving
Calories: 190 | Fat: 5 g | Protein: 2 g | Sodium: 40 mg
Fiber: 4 g | Carbohydrates: 37 g | Sugar: 22 g

APPLE PIE

Serves 2

INGREDIENTS

1 tablespoon apple cider vinegar
2 medium apples, cored and peeled
1 teaspoon cinnamon
1 cup rolled oats
1 cup ice
2 cups unsweetened vanilla almond milk

1 Combine all the ingredients in a large blender.

2 Blend the ingredients on high until thoroughly combined and frothy.

3 Consume immediately or store tightly sealed and unrefrigerated up to 4 hours.

KEY INGREDIENT: Apples

While apples are often used to add sweetness to dishes and desserts, there are also incredible benefits packed into every bite of these natural sweeties. Not only do apples of all varieties provide a number of vitamins, such as A, C, and B_6, and minerals, such as potassium and magnesium, but they are also full of antioxidants that protect cells from free radical damage. To sweeten the pot, apples contain massive amounts of fiber, which helps you achieve a feeling of fullness with a small amount of food. This same fibrous material helps cleanse the digestive system of waste byproducts that can interfere with bowel movements, inhibit proper nutrient absorption and distribution, and cause hormonal imbalances and metabolic fluctuations that can hinder weight loss. By including apples in your ACV drinks, you can be sure that you're getting the benefits of apples in their whole, natural state with the power of ACV's potency as well!

Per Serving
Calories: 250 | Fat: 7 g | Protein: 6 g | Sodium: 180 mg
Fiber: 7 g | Carbohydrates: 44 g | Sugar: 12 g

SLIMMING CITRUS

Serves 2

INGREDIENTS

1 tablespoon apple cider vinegar
1 medium pink grapefruit, peeled and deseeded
2 medium oranges, peeled and de-seeded
½ cup chopped pineapple
2 cups purified water (pH-balanced)

---

1 Combine all the ingredients in a large blender.

2 Blend the ingredients on high until thoroughly combined and frothy.

3 Consume immediately or store tightly sealed and unrefrigerated up to 4 hours.

KEY INGREDIENT: Grapefruit

Vitamin C plays a number of roles throughout the body. Not only does this essential vitamin protect against free radical damage, but it also boosts the immune system, supports proper metabolism, is essential for countless enzymatic activities, and promotes gut health. When you incorporate grapefruit into your day, you not only add sweet, slightly tart flavors to your culinary creations, but you also improve your body's health. When losing weight, it is absolutely imperative for the body's systems to work optimally and synergistically to ensure that everything from digestion to metabolic processes is firing as necessary. Contributing to sustained weight loss and healthy muscle and bone maintenance throughout life, grapefruit is both a sweet choice for your drinks and a wise one for your quality of life!

Per Serving
Calories: 120 | Fat: 0.5 g | Protein: 2 g | Sodium: 5 mg
Fiber: 5 g | Carbohydrates: 31 g | Sugar: 25 g

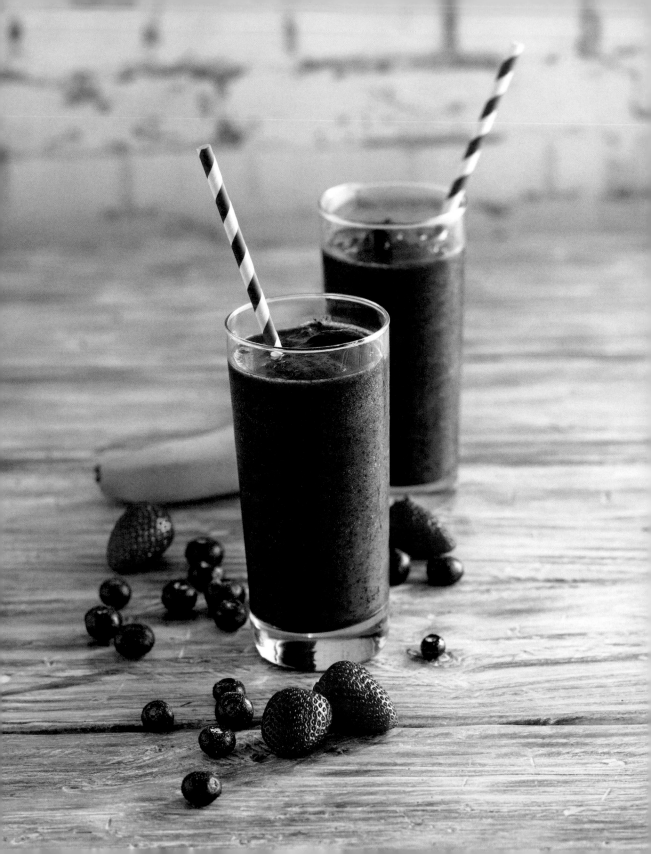

BERRIES AND BANANAS

Serves 2

INGREDIENTS

1 tablespoon apple cider vinegar
1 cup blueberries
1 cup hulled strawberries
2 medium bananas, peeled and
    frozen
1 cup ice
2 cups purified water (pH-balanced)

---

1 Combine all the ingredients in
    a large blender.

2 Blend the ingredients on high
    until thoroughly combined and
    frothy.

3 Consume immediately or store
    tightly sealed and unrefriger-
    ated up to 4 hours.

KEY INGREDIENT: Berries

While people tend to put all berries in the same category, each berry provides its own combination of vitamins, minerals, and antioxidants that promote health and well-being. For example, the anthocyanins in blueberries provide powerful antioxidant protection against free radical damage, and strawberries are renowned for providing more vitamin C than oranges. Berries are also filled with fiber and water, which both contribute to weight loss. Easily added to combinations that contain other sweet ingredients or even tart greens and unexpected additions, berries can balance flavors *and* provide outstanding nutrition. With just one serving of berries, such as blueberries or strawberries, a satisfying feeling of fullness can be achieved with the added bonus of plentiful energy and improved mental clarity. When these essential elements are mixed with all-powerful apple cider vinegar, sipping your way slim has never been easier.

Per Serving
Calories: 170 | Fat: 1 g | Protein: 2 g | Sodium: 5 mg
Fiber: 6 g | Carbohydrates: 43 g | Sugar: 25 g

Chapter 3

RECIPES FOR DETOXIFICATION

Whether you find yourself considering a detoxification program for removing impurities, improving overall health, or recovering from an overindulgent evening, there are a number of popular detox plans from which to choose. Many detox programs include drastic measures and intense restrictions, and while many of these detoxes seem to be effective, the harm done to the body can far outweigh the benefit. With adequate hydration and a clean diet of natural, nutrient-dense foods, such as fruits, vegetables, and additions, the body receives what it requires for optimal functioning. By adding apple cider vinegar to your diet, you can achieve detoxification throughout your entire body naturally. The enzymes and nutrients in ACV cleanse the blood, brain, cells, and organs of toxic substances and organisms, and support healthy maintenance and protection from future toxicity. Add the deliciousness of sweet fruits, antioxidant-rich produce, and other delectable additions, and you'll have a cleansing ACV creation that beats any other detox drink available!

LEMON-LIME MELON

Serves 2

INGREDIENTS

1 tablespoon apple cider vinegar

2 medium lemons, peeled and deseeded

2 medium limes, peeled and deseeded

1 cup chopped cantaloupe

1 tablespoon honey

2 cups purified water (pH-balanced)

---

1 Combine all the ingredients in
a large blender.

2 Blend the ingredients on high
until thoroughly combined and
frothy.

3 Consume immediately or store
tightly sealed and unrefrigerated up to 4 hours.

KEY INGREDIENT: Cantaloupe

In the process of detoxification, massive amounts of toxins can be released from the body; however, this can often leave your body in a critical state. While detoxifying, you need the support of nutrient-dense dietary elements that can help remove the toxins while also replenishing essential vitamins, minerals, and antioxidants. Cantaloupe, with its high water content, helps the body replenish essential nutrients while also hydrating the cells, organs, and systems in need. Cantaloupes are rich sources of vitamins A, C, B_6, and K, and minerals like potassium, calcium, iron, magnesium, phosphorus, and zinc. Cantaloupes also provide beta-carotene, which is converted to vitamin A, an essential nutrient that helps protect your cells from damage. The cantaloupe and ACV in this drink will ensure that every sip will help your body to detoxify while restoring and replenishing itself as well.

Per Serving
Calories: 90 | Fat: 0.5 g | Protein: 2 g | Sodium: 20 mg
Fiber: 4 g | Carbohydrates: 26 g | Sugar: 18 g

WATERMELON BASIL

Serves 2
INGREDIENTS

1 tablespoon apple cider vinegar
4 cups watermelon chunks
2 tablespoons chopped fresh basil
   leaves
1 cup ice
2 cups purified water (pH-balanced)

---

1 Combine all the ingredients in
   a large blender.

2 Blend the ingredients on high
   until thoroughly combined and
   frothy.

3 Consume immediately or store
   tightly sealed and unrefrigerated up to 4 hours.

KEY INGREDIENT: Basil

While herbs are not conventionally used in Western medicine, more and more people are turning to homeopathic herbal approaches to healing. Basil is just one of the aromatic herbs that not only add a delicious flavor to dishes and drinks but also provide an abundance of nutrients that both support the body's systems and detoxify at the same time. Basil's potent antioxidants surge through the digestive system and bloodstream, helping to purge the body of toxins and harmful agents. Delicious and nutritious, this delightful, light-tasting addition can transform the nutrition of a meal's ingredients while also improving the taste. Combine this herbaceous power with the benefits of ACV, and you've got a dream detox drink!

Per Serving
Calories: 90 | Fat: 0.5 g | Protein: 2 g | Sodium: 5 mg
Fiber: 1 g | Carbohydrates: 23 g | Sugar: 19 g

CUCUMBER MINT

Serves 2
INGREDIENTS

1 tablespoon apple cider vinegar
2 medium cucumbers, peeled and
   chopped
2 tablespoons fresh mint leaves
1 tablespoon honey
2 cups purified water (pH-balanced)

---

1 Combine all the ingredients in
   a large blender.

2 Blend the ingredients on high
   until thoroughly combined and
   frothy.

3 Consume immediately or store
   tightly sealed and unrefrigerated up to 4 hours.

KEY INGREDIENT: Cucumber

While many people consider cucumbers to be tasteless, the nutrition content and hydration qualities are quite overwhelming. A rich source of vitamin C, vitamin K, and minerals, such as silica, cucumbers can provide the body with restorative nutrients that not only support the detoxification process but also help to repair the body's systems that rely on these natural sources for support. In addition, cucumbers aid the digestive system by helping to cleanse the liver, the main detoxifying organ, by removing toxins and waste materials from the blood. Cucumbers are also a diuretic food, meaning they help the body produce more urine, which then carries out more toxins and waste. Because they help the cells, organs, and systems remain hydrated while toxins are purged, cucumbers are an essential addition to anyone's detoxification diet.

Per Serving
Calories: 60 | Fat: 0.5 g | Protein: 1 g | Sodium: 5 mg
Fiber: 2 g | Carbohydrates: 13 g | Sugar: 11 g

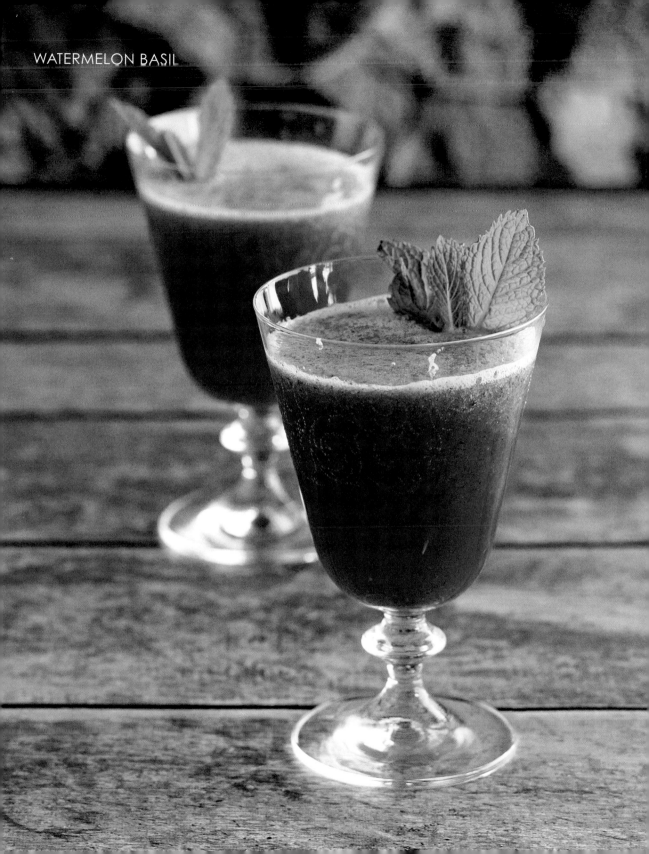

GINGER TEA TREAT

Serves 2
INGREDIENTS

1 tablespoon apple cider vinegar
2 cups green tea prepared with purified (pH-balanced) water, cooled
2 tablespoons peeled and grated
   fresh gingerroot
1 cup ice

---

1 Combine all the ingredients in
       a large blender.

2 Blend the ingredients on high
       until thoroughly combined and
       frothy.

3 Consume immediately or store
       tightly sealed and unrefriger-
       ated up to 4 hours.

KEY INGREDIENT: Green Tea

Antioxidants often receive attention for their abilities to combat free radical damage. Free radicals are unstable molecules that try to bond with other healthy molecules, thereby damaging them and causing aging, tissue damage, and certain diseases. The ability to fight free radicals makes antioxidant-rich foods and drinks some of the main staples in any detoxification program. Green tea is so rich in potent antioxidants that the inclusion of it in a detox program not only helps in the detoxification process but also promotes health and provides protection against the damaging free radicals. The addition of green tea—with its vitamins, minerals, and unique antioxidants called catechins—to drinks that also include apple cider vinegar can help restore a natural balance to the body for optimal health and successful detoxification. Simple to prepare, green tea can be made in large batches and stored in a refrigerator or freezer for an easy addition to delicious and nutritious detoxification recipes like this one.

Per Serving
Calories: 7 | Fat: 0 g | Protein: 1 g | Sodium: 5 mg
Fiber: 0 g | Carbohydrates: 1 g | Sugar: 0 g

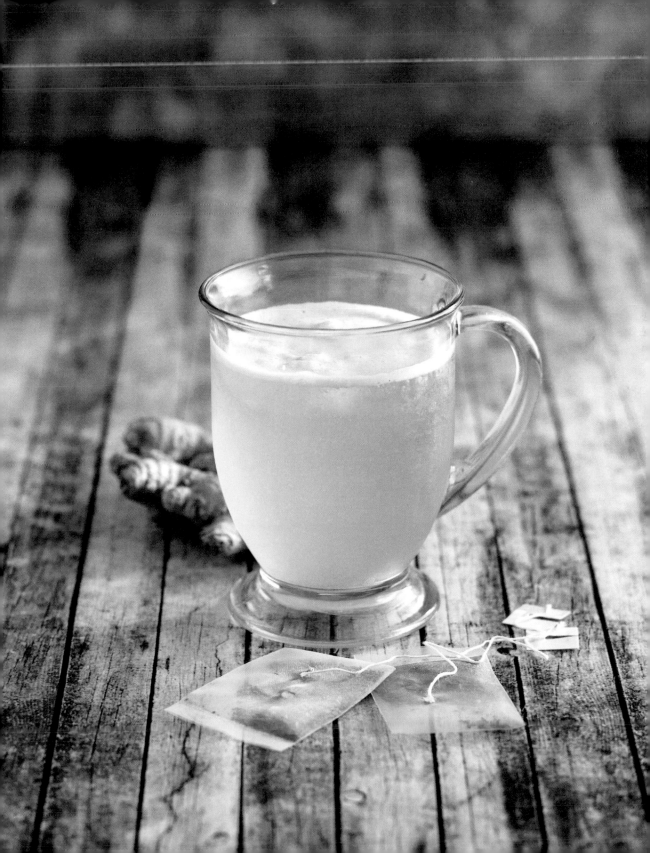

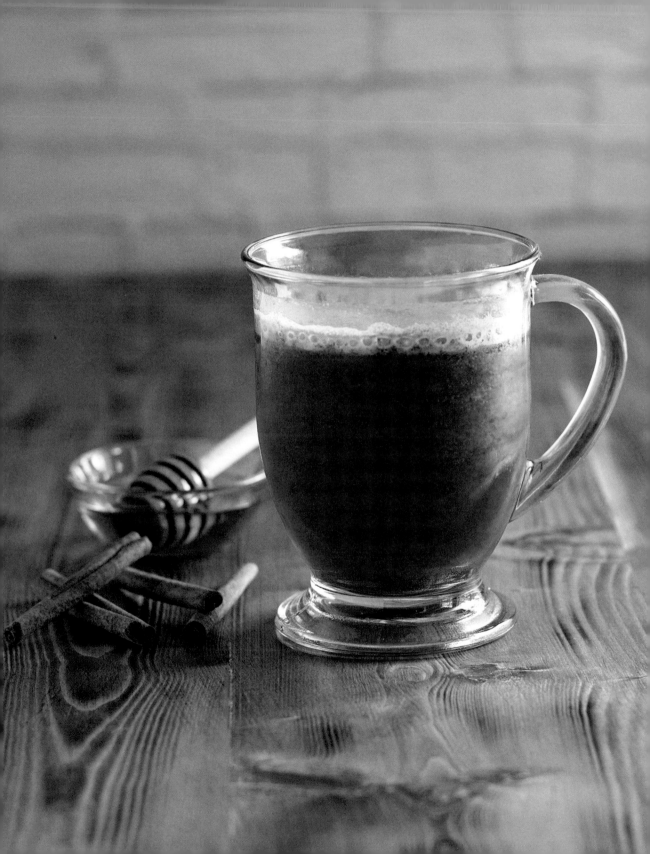

SPICED BLACK TEA WITH ACV

Serves 2

INGREDIENTS

1 tablespoon apple cider vinegar
2 cups black tea prepared with purified water (pH-balanced), cooled
1 tablespoon ground cinnamon
1 tablespoon ground cardamom
1 tablespoon honey
1 cup ice

1 Combine all the ingredients in
   a large blender.

2 Blend the ingredients on high
   until thoroughly combined
   and frothy.

3 Consume immediately or
   store tightly sealed and unrefrigerated up to 4 hours.

KEY INGREDIENT: Black Tea

While many teas are widely consumed for health reasons, black tea has received far less attention in this area than it truly deserves. Packed with plentiful antioxidants like polyphenols and catechins that help to purge the body of toxins and harmful free radicals while also restoring the natural health of the cells, organs, and systems, black tea is a simple ingredient that can be added to your diet for immense benefits. Recent studies also prove that drinking black tea can help lower LDL cholesterol and may be beneficial to people who have a high risk of heart disease. With delicious recipes like this one that combine this potent ingredient with apple cider vinegar's powerful enzymes, detoxification can be achieved quickly, easily, and naturally.

Per Serving
Calories: 50 | Fat: 0 g | Protein: 1 g | Sodium: 10 mg
Fiber: 3 g | Carbohydrates: 14 g | Sugar: 9 g

MASTER CLEANSE WITH ACV

Serves 2

INGREDIENTS

1 tablespoon apple cider vinegar
1 medium lemon, peeled and
  deseeded
1 tablespoon molasses
¼ teaspoon cayenne pepper
2 cups purified water (pH-balanced)

1 Combine all the ingredients in a large blender.

2 Blend the ingredients on high until thoroughly combined and frothy.

3 Consume immediately or store tightly sealed and unrefrigerated up to 4 hours.

KEY INGREDIENT: Cayenne Pepper

Cayenne pepper maximizes your detoxification program by revving up your metabolism, cleansing your blood, and boosting your energy for fat-burning workouts. Improving everything from cognitive functioning to digestion, cayenne pepper gets added to this delicious apple cider vinegar drink for maximized detoxification support. Helping to prevent illness with nutrients and potent phytochemicals (compounds found in plants that are believed to protect cells from cancer), cayenne pepper maximizes the detoxification process while also safeguarding against common issues associated with it, such as lack of energy and focus. Cayenne pepper can also help prevent the onset of illness that can occur when the immune system is compromised due to the nutrition-deficient diets commonly associated with detoxification. This spice is a real winner when it comes to delicious ACV drinks for detox. While the amount of cayenne pepper in this recipe may seem high, the amount added to this recipe can be adjusted depending upon your personal preference. The amount suggested is preferable, but any amount that allows for you to comfortably consume this drink is fine.

Per Serving
Calories: 40 | Fat: 0.5 g | Protein: 0 g | Sodium: 5 mg
Fiber: 1 g | Carbohydrates: 11 g | Sugar: 8 g

Chapter 4
RECIPES FOR BETTER DIGESTION

When digestive issues occur, the results can be catastrophic! Many people suffer from serious digestive discomfort on a regular basis, including pain, bloating, and embarrassing flatulence. Many digestive conditions can be effectively treated with over-the-counter or prescription medications, but some of these treatment methods contain questionable ingredients and synthetic additives that exacerbate digestive troubles. Each of the recipes in this chapter will help you better your digestion simply, easily, and naturally through the combination of whole, natural foods and apple cider vinegar. ACV contains important enzymes that support both the breakdown of foods and the absorption and utilization of nutrients that are required by the body. ACV also helps to regulate the pH of digestive juices and enzymes to ensure proper digestion of food, while also preventing overproduction of acidic bile that can back up into the esophagus. Swirled, shaken, or stirred into delicious combinations of stomach-soothing foods, ACV can help alleviate some the most disruptive digestive issues.

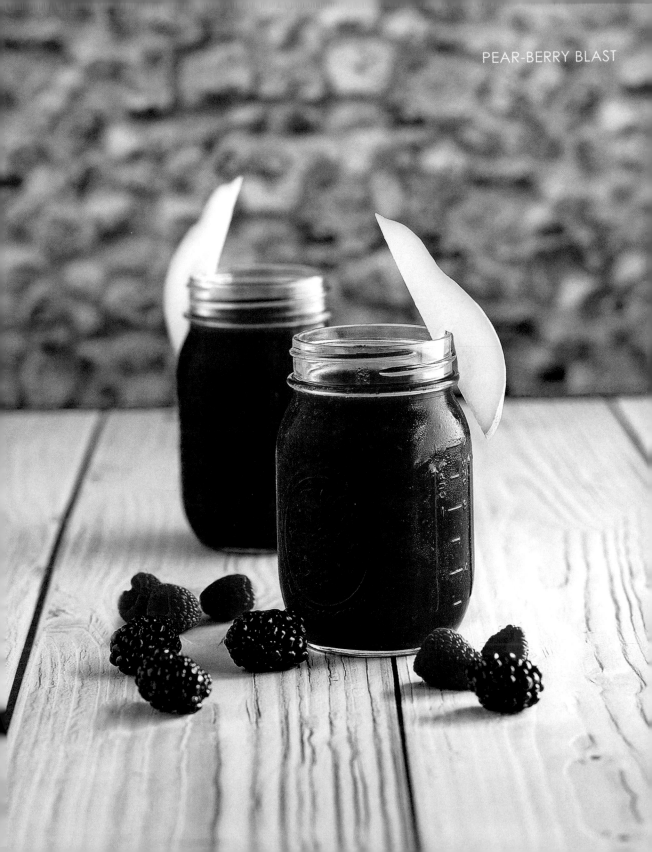

PEAR-BERRY BLAST

Serves 2
INGREDIENTS

1 tablespoon apple cider vinegar
1 medium pear, peeled and cored
1 cup raspberries
1 cup blackberries
2 cups purified water (pH-balanced)

1   Combine all the ingredients in a large blender.
2   Blend the ingredients on high until thoroughly combined and frothy.
3   Consume immediately or store tightly sealed and unrefrigerated up to 4 hours.

KEY INGREDIENT: Pears

With plentiful vitamins and minerals, such as vitamins A, C, and K, iron, magnesium, and phosphorus, pears provide gut-friendly fiber that aids in digestion. Fiber helps ferry food through the digestive system without the fear of food particles being caught in the large intestine's pockets. Apple cider vinegar assists in this work by providing nutritious enzymes that help break down food as it passes through the digestive system. Improving digestion and supporting the body by ensuring the proper absorption and distribution of nutrients, pears and ACV combine to create the perfect drink for digestion!

Per Serving
Calories: 100 | Fat: 1 g | Protein: 2 g | Sodium: 4 mg
Fiber: 10 g | Carbohydrates: 25 g | Sugar: 13 g

YOGURT-BERRY BLAST

Serves 2
INGREDIENTS

1 tablespoon apple cider vinegar
1 cup nonfat plain Greek yogurt
1 cup blueberries
1 cup hulled strawberries
1 cup ice
1 cup purified water (pH-balanced)

1   Combine all the ingredients in a large blender.
2   Blend the ingredients on high until thoroughly combined and frothy.
3   Consume immediately or store tightly sealed and refrigerated up to 4 hours.

KEY INGREDIENT: Greek Yogurt

Yogurt is a common ingredient found in many different kinds of recipes, from smoothies and sauces to breads and baked goods. If you're accustomed to the traditional creamy version, consider giving the thick Greek variety a try. Like regular yogurt, Greek yogurt is made by adding bacterial cultures to milk and then allowing it to ferment. With Greek yogurt there's an extra step: the yogurt is strained to remove liquid, whey, and lactose, resulting in a thicker yogurt. In addition to packing in plentiful protein, Greek yogurt is also renowned for its powerful probiotics. These probiotics not only promote healthy digestion but also maintain a proper bacteria balance that assists in the breakdown of foods and distribution of nutrients throughout the body.

Per Serving
Calories: 130 | Fat: 1 g | Protein: 13 g | Sodium: 45 mg
Fiber: 3 g | Carbohydrates: 20 g | Sugar: 14 g

KALE CARROT APPLE

Serves 2

INGREDIENTS

1 tablespoon apple cider vinegar

2 large kale leaves with ribs removed, chopped

2 medium carrots, peeled and chopped

1 large Fuji apple, peeled and cored

2 cups purified water (pH-balanced)

---

1 Combine all the ingredients in a large blender.

2 Blend the ingredients on high until thoroughly combined and frothy.

3 Consume immediately or store tightly sealed and unrefrigerated up to 4 hours.

KEY INGREDIENT: Kale

Kale is an amazing ingredient to be included in any diet focused on digestive improvement or overall health. This healthy green has ample amounts of vitamin K, which supports the body's processing of essential nutrients, such as iron and calcium. In addition, kale's fiber helps ensure that bits of undigested debris are moved through the digestive system without issue. While many people who are new to kale may experience a "cleansing" effect that involves more bathroom trips than normally required, this green leafy vegetable provides more help than harm in countless ways, including digestive function, nutrient absorption, and nutrient availability to the cells, organs, and systems.

Per Serving

Calories: 120 | Fat: 1 g | Protein: 3 g | Sodium: 65 mg
Fiber: 6 g | Carbohydrates: 26 g | Sugar: 16 g

CREAMY CITRUS SURPRISE

Serves 2

INGREDIENTS

1 tablespoon apple cider vinegar

2 medium oranges, peeled and deseeded

½ cup chopped pineapple

½ medium grapefruit, peeled and deseeded

1 cup ice

2 cups low-fat plain Greek yogurt

1 Combine all the ingredients in a large blender.

2 Blend the ingredients on high until thoroughly combined and frothy.

3 Consume immediately or store tightly sealed and refrigerated up to 4 hours.

KEY INGREDIENT: Pineapple

Pineapple is a powerhouse when it comes to your health. Its plentiful stores of vitamin C and the mineral manganese work as antioxidants, protecting against cell damage caused by free radicals, and manganese also assists with energy production. But pineapple is especially great for digestion, from relieving indigestion to assisting with more serious digestive issues, such as irritable bowel syndrome and diverticulosis. This is due to the presence of an enzyme called bromelain, which helps your body break down and absorb proteins from the food you eat. With supportive benefits and a uniquely tangy taste, pineapple makes for the perfect accompaniment to apple cider vinegar in this delicious and nutritious drink.

Per Serving

Calories: 270 | Fat: 5 g | Protein: 24 g | Sodium: 80 mg
Fiber: 4 g | Carbohydrates: 35 g | Sugar: 29 g

PEACH-CHERRY CRUMBLE

Serves 2

INGREDIENTS

1 tablespoon apple cider vinegar
1 medium peach, pitted
1 cup pitted cherries
¼ cup rolled oats
1 teaspoon ground cinnamon
1 cup ice
2 cups unsweetened almond milk

1   Combine all the ingredients in a large blender.

2   Blend the ingredients on high until thoroughly combined and frothy.

3   Consume immediately or store tightly sealed and either refrigerated or unrefrigerated up to 4 hours.

KEY INGREDIENT: Oats

While carbohydrates, such as grains, are notorious for causing weight gain, there are certain varieties of whole grains that help with weight loss, detoxification, and digestion. Oats are the perfect example because they provide essential nutrients, which encourage healthy, sustained energy production, as well as filling fiber, which aids in digestive system processes. Oats contain both soluble and insoluble fiber. When combined with water, soluble fiber forms a gel-like substance that moves slowly through the digestive system, delaying digestion of food. This slow pace allows your body to absorb more nutrients through the intestinal walls while also delaying sugar absorption. Insoluble fiber, on the other hand, acts as a scrub brush, cleaning out your bowels. In addition, the fiber in oats helps to maintain the optimal health of the digestive system by boosting good bacteria in your gut while keeping harmful bacteria at safe levels. Oats and apple cider vinegar work hand in hand in this recipe to keep the digestive system and the immune system in good working order.

Per Serving
Calories: 160 | Fat: 4 g | Protein: 4 g | Sodium: 190 mg
Fiber: 4 g | Carbohydrates: 29 g | Sugar: 16 g

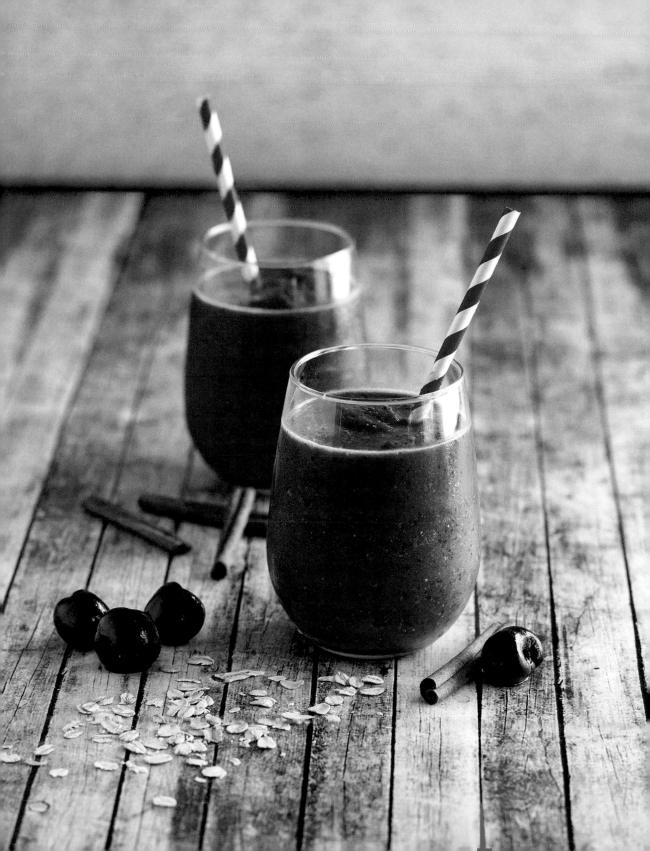

GINGER-APPLE CREAM

Serves 2

INGREDIENTS

1 tablespoon apple cider vinegar

1 tablespoon peeled and grated fresh gingerroot

2 medium Pink Lady apples, peeled and cored

2 cups nonfat vanilla Greek yogurt

1 cup ice

½ cup purified water (pH-balanced)

---

1 Combine all the ingredients in a large blender.

2 Blend the ingredients on high until thoroughly combined and frothy.

3 Consume immediately or store tightly sealed and refrigerated up to 4 hours.

KEY INGREDIENT: Ginger

For centuries ginger has been heralded as a potent natural ingredient for digestive remedies. Easily peeled and grated, shredded, or juiced, ginger provides compounds called gingerols that ease stomachaches, aid in digestive processes, and assist with the proper processing of digestive enzymes that can be compromised by the standard American diet of fatty, fried, and sugary foods. When combined with apple cider vinegar, ginger's chemical components provide the body with naturally soothing remedies that relieve negative fluctuations in the body's synchronistic processes and aid in digestion. Natural, sweet, and slightly spicy, ginger adds a delightful element, taste-wise and nutrition-wise, to any ACV drink designed for digestive support.

Per Serving
Calories: 250 | Fat: 0.5 g | Protein: 20 g | Sodium: 80 mg
Fiber: 5 g | Carbohydrates: 43 g | Sugar: 35 g

SWEET SPIRULINA AND SPINACH

Serves 2

INGREDIENTS

1 teaspoon apple cider vinegar
¼ teaspoon spirulina
1 medium pear, peeled and cored
1 medium banana, peeled
1 tablespoon honey
2 cups spinach leaves
1 cup ice
2 cups chamomile tea prepared
    with purified water (pH-balanced),
    chilled

---

1 Combine all the ingredients in
    a large blender.

2 Blend the ingredients on high
    until thoroughly combined and
    frothy.

3 Consume immediately or store
    tightly sealed and unrefriger-
    ated up to 4 hours.

KEY INGREDIENT: Spinach

While raw spinach is often considered the star of a simple salad plate, this nutritious deep-green leafy veggie can be added to a variety of dishes and drinks without altering the flavor. With that in mind, many people have started incorporating spinach leaves into their smoothies, shakes, and snacks to boost their nutritional content while maintaining the flavor of their favorite culinary creations. For people who struggle with digestive issues, the benefits of spinach run deep. It regulates pH—which provides alkaline benefits to the acids and enzymes in the stomach that cause indigestion—and has an abundance of fiber that cleanses the colon of undigested food particles and debris that can get trapped in the pockets of the intestinal walls and cause chronic pain and discomfort. Combined with ACV's enzymes that promote gut health, prevent infection, and reduce inflammation, spinach makes for the perfect ACV drink addition for anyone in need of digestive health improvement.

Per Serving
Calories: 130 | Fat: 0.5 g | Protein: 2 g | Sodium: 35 mg
Fiber: 4 g | Carbohydrates: 34 g | Sugar: 23 g

GREEN APPLE

Serves 2

INGREDIENTS

1 tablespoon apple cider vinegar

1 cup spinach leaves

2 medium Granny Smith apples,
   peeled and cored

1 tablespoon ground cinnamon

1 teaspoon ground nutmeg

¼ teaspoon ground cloves

1 tablespoon honey

1 cup ice

2 cups purified water (pH-balanced)

---

1 Combine all the ingredients in
a large blender.

2 Blend the ingredients on high
until thoroughly combined and
frothy.

3 Consume immediately or store
tightly sealed and unrefrigerated up to 4 hours.

KEY INGREDIENT: Spinach

Rich in iron and vitamin K as well as folate and fiber, spinach is the perfect food for digestive health. Cups of this leafy
green vegetable can be added to almost any dish or drink
without drastically altering the desired taste of the main
ingredients. Ample amounts of antioxidants support the
health-amplifying effects of spinach by boosting the body's
natural protection of cells, organs, and systems against the
barrage of free radical damage you encounter every day.
Vitamins, minerals, and potent phytochemicals are all added
to your favorite delicious and nutritious apple cider vinegar
drinks when spinach is included. With no bitter taste and
with plentiful benefits, spinach is a fantastic option for anyone hoping to promote their digestive health.

Per Serving
Calories: 130 | Fat: 1 g | Protein: 1 g | Sodium: 15 mg
Fiber: 7 g | Carbohydrates: 32 g | Sugar: 22 g

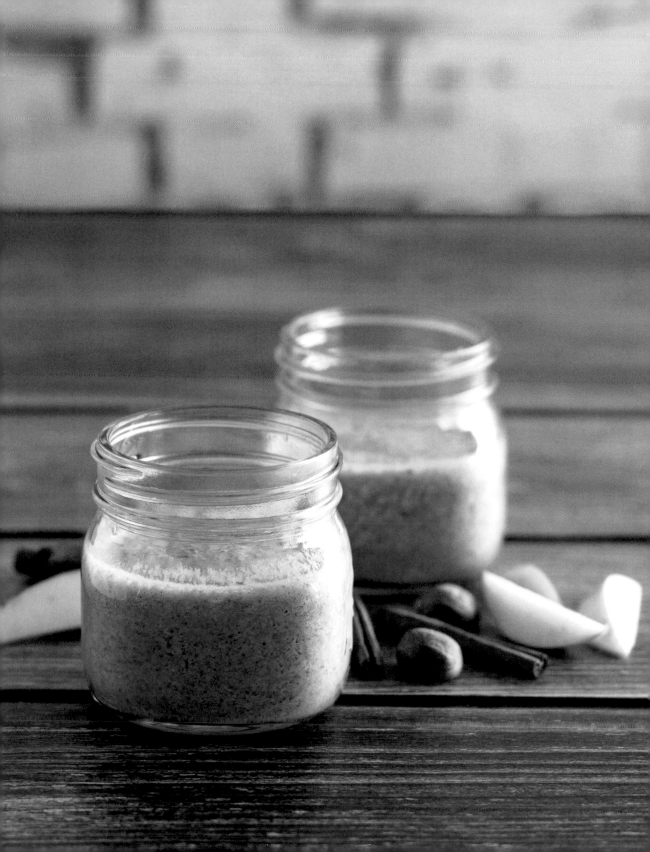

Chapter 5

RECIPES FOR COLD AND SINUS RELIEF

Colds, flus, and sinus-related conditions can strike at any time, regardless of the season. As a result, consumers purchase an astounding number of over-the-counter medicines with the hope of minimizing or eliminating the associated symptoms while the body fights the illness. While it can be tempting to pop a pill or swig a syrup that claims to relieve the pain, pressure, and discomfort that colds and sinus issues can cause, the hidden dangers of these often ineffective remedies, such as harsh chemicals and additives, can outweigh the benefits. Luckily, for centuries apple cider vinegar has been shown to minimize the effects and duration of colds and eliminate the underlying causes of sinus issues and infections. With antibacterial, antiviral, and antimicrobial benefits, ACV provides the body with an all-natural healing approach that helps strengthen the immune system while fighting the illness quickly and effectively. In this chapter, apple cider vinegar stars in some of the most amazingly effective and delectable drinks that cleanse the body of illness-causing microbes, bacteria, and viruses while providing the body with natural nutrition from vibrant whole foods.

SWEET AND SPICY GINGER-MELON

Serves 2
INGREDIENTS

- 1 tablespoon apple cider vinegar
- 2 tablespoons peeled and grated fresh gingerroot
- 1 cup chopped cantaloupe
- 1 cup chopped honeydew
- 2 cups chamomile tea prepared with purified water (pH-balanced), chilled

1 Combine all the ingredients in a large blender.

2 Blend the ingredients on high until thoroughly combined and frothy.

3 Consume immediately or store tightly sealed and unrefrigerated up to 4 hours.

KEY INGREDIENT: Chamomile Tea

Chamomile is an aromatic plant in the daisy family. Chamomile tea contains small amounts of calcium, magnesium, potassium, folate, and vitamin A, but its true health benefits come from its flavonoids. Flavonoids are a group of phytonutrients (plant chemicals) that have powerful anti-inflammatory and immune system benefits. Chamomile tea also possesses antimicrobial and antioxidant properties. In addition, this noncaffeinated beverage will rehydrate you, is ideal for flushing bacteria out of your system, and is well known as a sleep aid, which will give your body time to heal itself and kick your cold. With essential nutrients and protective phytochemicals that help calm the mind and fight infection, the combination of ACV and chamomile tea makes for an easy-to-make concoction that can be steeped and kept refrigerated in large batches for quick cold relief. Delicious and crisp, this is the perfect preparation to be consumed at the onset of illness, after the cold or sinus infection has developed, or even for future prevention after the illness has passed.

Per Serving
Calories: 60 | Fat: 0.5 g | Protein: 1 g | Sodium: 35 mg
Fiber: 2 g | Carbohydrates: 16 g | Sugar: 13 g

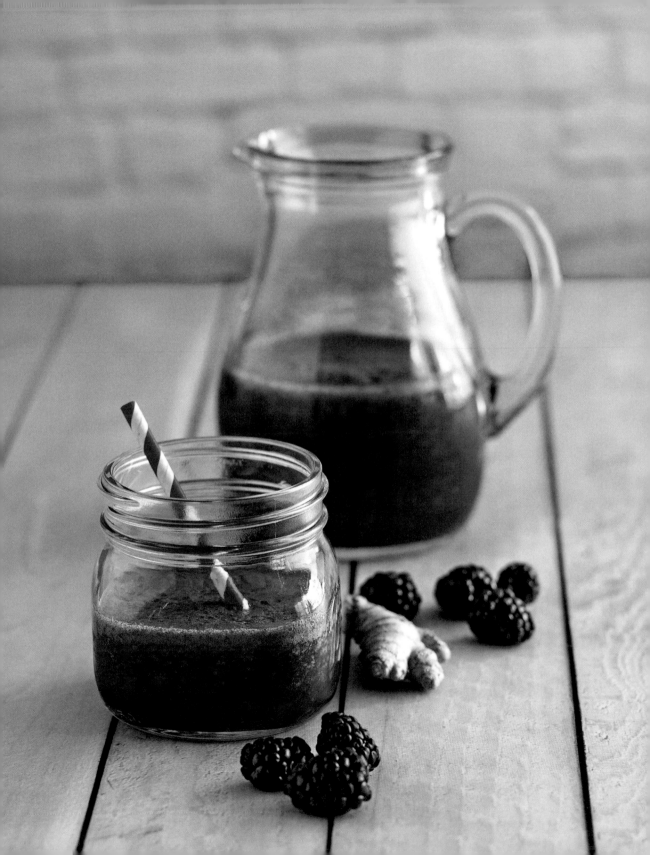

BLACKBERRY TEA

Serves 2

INGREDIENTS

1 tablespoon apple cider vinegar

2 cups blackberries

1 medium banana, peeled and frozen

1 teaspoon peeled and grated fresh gingerroot

1 cup ice

2 cups black tea prepared with purified water (pH-balanced), chilled

1 Combine all the ingredients in a large blender.

2 Blend the ingredients on high until thoroughly combined and frothy.

3 Consume immediately or store tightly sealed and unrefrigerated up to 4 hours.

KEY INGREDIENT: Blackberries

Few people are aware of the plentiful benefits blackberries can provide when dealing with respiratory disruptions. Blackberries are high in magnesium and vitamin C; contain polyphenols that are associated with fighting cold and flu, like vitamin E does; and possess plentiful antioxidants. These berries also contain a significant amount of iron, which naturally boosts your immunity by increasing your hemoglobin and oxygen concentrations in the blood. This increases your body's ability to fight off infections, prevent colds and flu, and stave off bacteria and viruses. The ample amounts of vitamin C in blackberries combine with apple cider vinegar's powerful enzymes to support the body's natural abilities to combat colds, flus, bacterial infections, viral infections, and microbial combatants that wreak havoc on the immune system. Along with ACV, blackberries provide the body and mind with essential nutrition and also taste delicious.

Per Serving

Calories: 120 | Fat: 1 g | Protein: 3 g | Sodium: 10 mg
Fiber: 9 g | Carbohydrates: 28 g | Sugar: 14 g

SPICED HONEY-GINGER TEA

Serves 2

INGREDIENTS

1 tablespoon apple cider vinegar

2 cups white tea prepared with purified water (pH-balanced), chilled

1 tablespoon peeled and grated
fresh gingerroot

¼ teaspoon ground cloves

1 Combine all the ingredients in
a large blender.

2 Blend the ingredients on high
until thoroughly combined and
frothy.

3 Consume immediately or store
tightly sealed and unrefrigerated up to 4 hours.

KEY INGREDIENT: Cloves

Cloves are the dried flower buds of the clove tree, which can be used in whole or ground form. This aromatic spice provides the body with immune system support that helps to protect against and prevent illness. Cloves contain calcium, iron, magnesium, potassium, riboflavin, niacin, folate, and vitamins C, B_{12}, A, E, D, and K among others. Cloves have antibacterial and pain-killing properties, and are well known to help boost the immune system by increasing the white blood cell count. Cloves act to repair free radical damage and support healthy cell functioning. Cloves also alleviate inflammation that can result from, or contribute to, discomfort and disease. By combining cloves with ACV, anyone suffering from the common cold, flu, or sinus-related illnesses can find relief in an all-natural mixture that not only tastes great but also supports all of the body's systems and maintains overall health. Delicious and nutritious, this combination of ingredients makes for a sweet and spicy answer to any sinus sufferer's prayers!

Per Serving
Calories: 3 | Fat: 0 g | Protein: 0 g | Sodium: 15 mg
Fiber: 0 g | Carbohydrates: 1 g | Sugar: 0 g

GINGER-INFUSED GREEN TEA

Serves 4

INGREDIENTS

4 cups purified water (pH-balanced)
4 organic green tea bags
2 tablespoons peeled and sliced fresh
gingerroot
4 tablespoons apple cider vinegar

1 Bring water to a boil and remove from heat.

2 Add green tea bags and sliced ginger, cover, and allow to steep 4–8 hours.

3 Pour 4 equal (1-cup) portions of tea and add 1 tablespoon of ACV to each. Shake vigorously or blend on high to combine.

4 Consume immediately or store tightly sealed and unrefrigerated up to 4 hours.

KEY INGREDIENT: Apple Cider Vinegar

The enzymatic reactions from "the mother" of apple cider vinegar help to support cell health, assist in organ function, and maintain proper system processes for optimal overall health. In terms of sinus infection and cold prevention, ACV provides antimicrobial, antibacterial, antifungal, and antiviral support that helps protect against the onset of all types of illness. In addition, apple cider vinegar can help thin the mucus that often comes with sinus infections or irritations. While supporting the immune system, ACV protects against the illnesses and conditions that can contribute to sinus irritation, respiratory infection, and airway constriction.

Per Serving
Calories: 0 | Fat: 0 g | Protein: 0 g | Sodium: 0 mg
Fiber: 0 g | Carbohydrates: 0 g | Sugar: 0 g

SPICED SPINACH SMOOTHIE

Serves 2

INGREDIENTS

1 tablespoon apple cider vinegar

2 cups spinach leaves

1 medium Granny Smith apple, peeled and cored

1 tablespoon peeled and grated fresh gingerroot

1 cup ice

2 cups purified water (pH-balanced)

1 Combine all the ingredients in a large blender.

2 Blend the ingredients on high until thoroughly combined and frothy.

3 Consume immediately or store tightly sealed and unrefrigerated up to 4 hours.

KEY INGREDIENT: Ginger

Ginger contains unique compounds called gingerols that provide protection against illness. These gingerols act as potent antioxidants, combining with the enzymes and nutrients of apple cider vinegar to provide the body with defense against the common cold. Ginger helps to treat colds in several ways: it contains antiviral properties that fight against bacteria and illness, it contains antiseptic and anti-inflammatory properties that boost the immune system, it acts as a cough suppressant, it stimulates perspiration to bring down the body temperature, and it is a natural pain reliever. A cold or sinus infection sufferer can be tricked into buying over-the-counter cold and sinus medications that treat symptoms but leave the underlying cause of the condition unresolved. Additionally, these medications are often packed with chemicals, additives, and harsh synthetics that can actually weaken the body. With ginger and ACV, this drink becomes a delicious alternative promising protection and prevention.

Per Serving
Calories: 50 | Fat: 0.5 g | Protein: 1 g | Sodium: 25 mg
Fiber: 3 g | Carbohydrates: 11 g | Sugar: 7 g

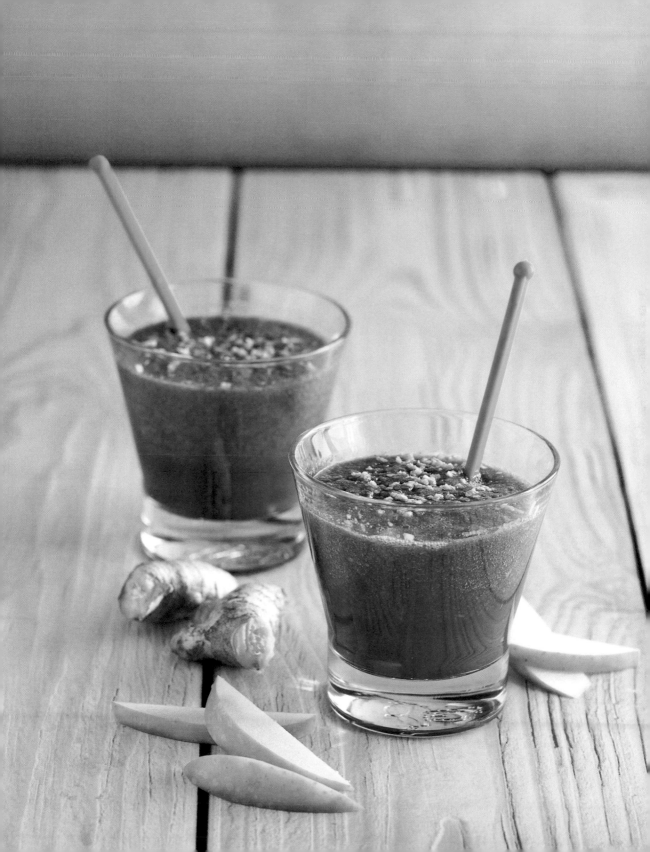

SWEET SPICY CITRUS

Serves 2

INGREDIENTS

1 tablespoon apple cider vinegar

1 tablespoon honey

1 medium orange, peeled and deseeded

1 medium lemon, peeled and deseeded

1 cup chopped pineapple

½ tablespoon deseeded and minced jalapeño

1 cup ice

2 cups purified water (pH-balanced)

---

1 Combine all the ingredients in a large blender.

2 Blend the ingredients on high until thoroughly combined and frothy.

3 Consume immediately or store tightly sealed and unrefrigerated up to 4 hours.

KEY INGREDIENT: Jalapeño

If you like spicy food but find yourself suffering from a cold, you're in luck. The compound that is responsible for the jalapeño's fiery flavor, capsaicin, also increases metabolic functions to heat the body, creating a "burning" effect that combats viruses like the common cold. Studies have shown that capsaicin reduces sinus symptoms such as nasal congestion, runny nose, sneezing, coughing, and mucus production. As capsaicin combines with the enzymes in apple cider vinegar, it helps your body's systems fight the infections that can plague the respiratory system and sinuses with irritation and inflammation. When dealing with a cold, flu, or sinus infection, the combination of ACV and the jalapeño's vitamins, minerals, and naturally occurring phytochemicals can help clear the airways, fend off infection, and improve the overall health of the entire body.

Per Serving

Calories: 110 | Fat: 0.5 g | Protein: 1 g | Sodium: 4 mg
Fiber: 4 g | Carbohydrates: 29 g | Sugar: 23 g

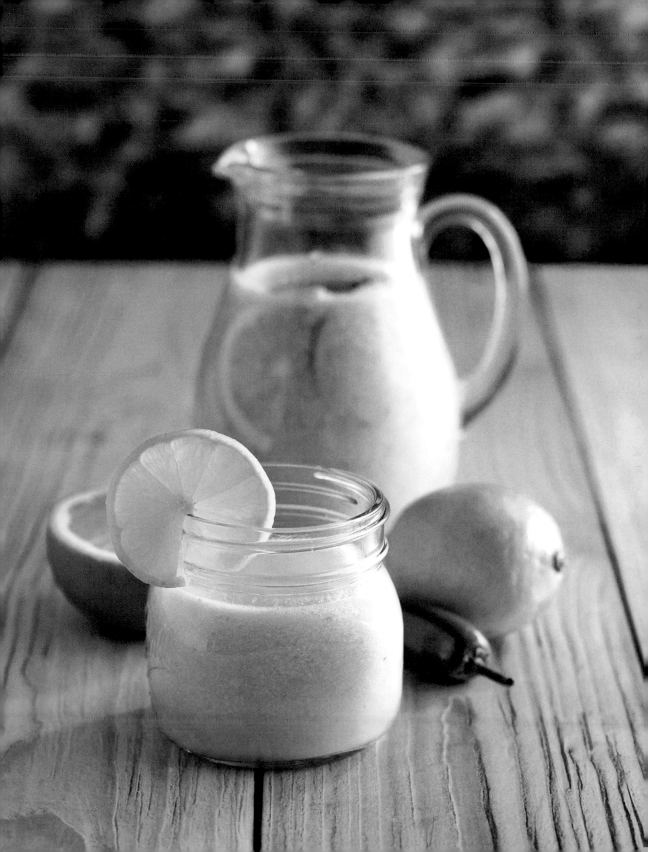

GARLIC GAZPACHO

Serves 2

INGREDIENTS

1 tablespoon apple cider vinegar
2 cloves garlic, peeled
½ medium white onion, peeled and
   chopped
2 large tomatoes, halved
1 tablespoon fresh cilantro leaves
2 cups purified water (pH-balanced)

1 Combine all the ingredients in
   a large blender.

2 Blend the ingredients on high
   until thoroughly combined and
   frothy.

3 Consume immediately or store
   tightly sealed and unrefrigerated up to 4 hours.

KEY INGREDIENT: Garlic

Garlic is known for helping to alleviate sinus infection symp-toms and protecting against illness. Garlic can be used as an all-natural and effective treatment for chronic inflamma-tion that surpasses the effectiveness and safety of the over-the-counter and prescription alternatives. When combined with apple cider vinegar, garlic's allicin helps to promote the immune system's functioning by ensuring that viruses and bacterial and microbial invaders are kept at bay. With the additional power to prevent free radical damage to cells, gar-lic's phytochemicals and ACV's enzymes combine to protect the immune system against the degradation that can lead to chronic conditions and serious illness. Delicious and nutri-tious, this savory drink makes sinus relief and cold preven-tion quick, easy, and tasty.

Per Serving
Calories: 48 | Fat: 0.5 g | Protein: 2 g | Sodium: 15 mg
Fiber: 3 g | Carbohydrates: 11 g | Sugar: 6 g

Chapter 6

RECIPES FOR HEALTHY SKIN AND HAIR

Every year, the hair and skin care industries generate billions of dollars. With pills, potions, creams, and oils that promise to leave skin feeling firm and wrinkle-free, or hair shiny, voluminous, and easy to manage, these industries guarantee to fix almost every flaw imaginable. While the marketing can be creative and the advertised results enticing, many of these products are costly, contain chemicals, and fail to produce the desired effects. Because the roots of beautiful hair and skin come from within, the focus should be on what you put *into* your body, not what you put *onto* it. Through a diet rich in protein, vitamin E, and antioxidant-packed whole foods, anyone can achieve more beautiful hair and skin naturally by simply providing the body with the essentials for healthy functioning. Adding apple cider vinegar and its supportive enzymes and nutrients to your diet can also help detoxify and cleanse your body of impurities, leading to healthier hair and skin. With this chapter's delectable drinks, you can sip your way to supple skin and lustrous locks healthfully, naturally, and deliciously!

ALOE VERA BLUE BANANA

Serves 2

INGREDIENTS

1 tablespoon apple cider vinegar
1 cup aloe vera juice
1 cup blueberries
1 medium banana, peeled and frozen
2 cups purified water (pH-balanced)

1 Combine all the ingredients in a large blender.

2 Blend the ingredients on high until thoroughly combined and frothy.

3 Consume immediately or store tightly sealed and unrefrigerated up to 4 hours.

KEY INGREDIENT: Banana

Packed with potassium, fiber, magnesium, manganese, and vitamins A, B$_6$, and C, creamy bananas make apple cider vinegar drinks like this one even more delicious and nutritious. The antioxidants and manganese in bananas protect the body from free radical damage, which can lead to premature aging of the skin. The vitamin A in bananas can help restore lost moisture in skin and can aid in repairing damaged or dry skin. Bananas also contain the mineral silica, which is thought to improve hair health and thickness. Helping to maintain a healthy balance of nutrients and essential moisture within the skin's cells and the hair's strands, bananas and ACV work hand in hand to ensure that all of the body's nutrient needs are met with extra enzymes and supportive phytochemicals for maximized benefits. ACV drinks that include all-natural fruits, like bananas, can meet and even exceed the body's nutritional needs.

Per Serving
Calories: 100 | Fat: 0.5 g | Protein: 1 g | Sodium: 30 mg
Fiber: 3 g | Carbohydrates: 26 g | Sugar: 14 g

BERRY NUTTY CREAMY CREATION

Serves 2

INGREDIENTS

1 tablespoon apple cider vinegar
1 cup blueberries
1 cup raspberries
1 cup raw whole almonds
1 cup ice
2 cups low-fat plain Greek yogurt

1 Combine all the ingredients in a large blender.

2 Blend the ingredients on high until thoroughly combined and frothy.

3 Consume immediately or store tightly sealed and refrigerated up to 4 hours.

KEY INGREDIENT: Almonds

Loaded with protein and vitamin E, almonds provide essential nutrition for achieving amazing skin and beautiful hair. When you have ample amounts of protein in your diet, your body is able to process nutrients and perform systematic functions that work to boost the appearance and health of your skin and hair. Vitamin E, a powerful antioxidant, combats cell damage caused by free radicals that can show up in these parts of your body. The combination of nutrient-packed almonds and enzyme-rich ACV keeps the body and mind healthy and promotes the growth and health of hair and skin.

Per Serving
Calories: 650 | Fat: 41 g | Protein: 39 g | Sodium: 80 mg
Fiber: 15 g | Carbohydrates: 42 g | Sugar: 21 g

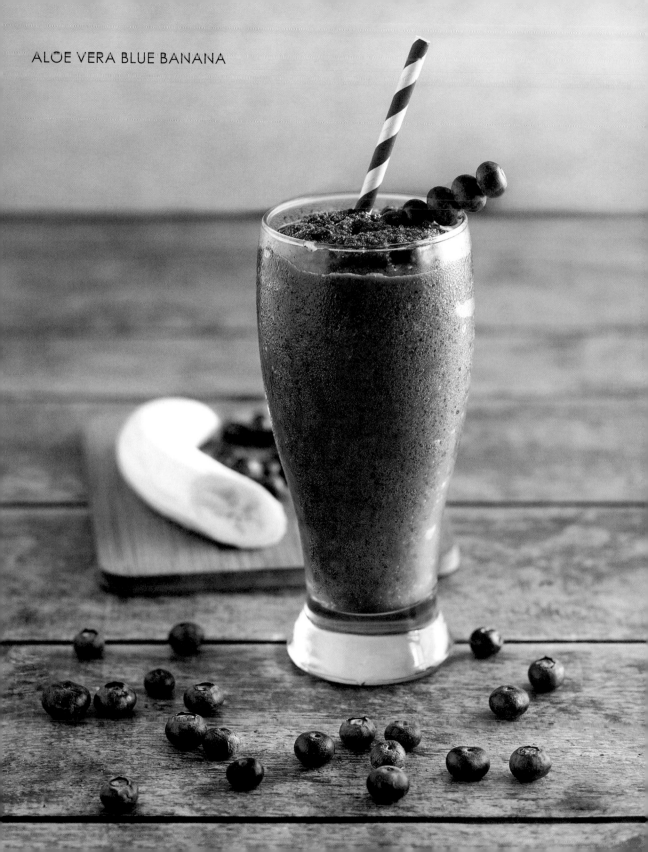

ALOE VERA BLUE BANANA

ALOE VERA KIWI CREAM

Serves 2

INGREDIENTS

1 tablespoon apple cider vinegar
2 medium kiwis, peeled
1 medium cucumber, peeled and
    chopped
½ cup food-grade aloe vera gel
1 cup nonfat plain Greek yogurt
1 cup ice
1 cup purified water (pH-balanced)

1 Combine all the ingredients in
   a large blender.

2 Blend the ingredients on high
   until thoroughly combined and
   frothy.

3 Consume immediately or store
   tightly sealed and refrigerated
   up to 4 hours.

KEY INGREDIENT: Aloe Vera

Aloe vera gel is the clear jellylike substance found in the inner part of the aloe vera leaf. More than seventy-five active components have been identified in aloe vera, including vitamins A, C, and E; folic acid; choline; minerals such as copper, calcium, manganese, potassium, and zinc; amino acids; enzymes; and salicylic acids. Aloe vera provides twenty of the twenty-two amino acids required by humans, including eight of the essential amino acids. Aloe vera has amazing nourishing properties and anti-inflammatory agents; it has the ability to speed the healing of wounds; and its antioxidants fight free radical damage to the skin and hair. With plentiful vitamins, minerals, and phytochemicals that provide the body with healing nutrition, aloe vera can be consumed for wide-ranging health benefits. Working to restore balance to hormone levels, replenish the cells with essential nutrition, and fortify the body's natural healing processes, aloe vera can be combined with apple cider vinegar to create the perfect combination of restorative nutrients that improve the condition of the skin and hair naturally. Aloe vera maintains and improves the body's natural immune defenses, maximizes nutrient absorption and distribution in the body, and helps to retain moisture in the cells. Aloe vera combines with ACV to ensure that the body has the essential proteins, fats, and nutrients that make hair healthy and shiny and cause the skin to glow.

Per Serving
Calories: 130 | Fat: 1 g | Protein: 13 g | Sodium: 75 mg
Fiber: 3 g | Carbohydrates: 18 g | Sugar: 12 g

CREAMY NUTS AND HONEY

Serves 2

INGREDIENTS

1 tablespoon apple cider vinegar
1½ cups low-fat vanilla Greek yogurt
½ cup walnuts
½ cup almonds
1 tablespoon honey
1 cup ice
1 cup purified water (pH-balanced)

---

1 Combine all the ingredients, except the water, in a large blender.

2 Blend the ingredients on high until thoroughly combined and frothy.

3 Add the water gradually and continue blending until desired consistency is reached.

4 Consume immediately or store tightly sealed and refrigerated up to 4 hours.

KEY INGREDIENT: Greek Yogurt

While many varieties of yogurt promise to provide essential nutrition, the majority of the commonly consumed brands contain little nourishment and unhealthy amounts of sugar. This added sugar can come with heavy costs, such as compromising the immune system, detracting from the nutrition that could otherwise be consumed in healthier meals and snacks, and interfering with the body's natural processing of essential nutrients. Greek yogurt, on the other hand, contains less sugar and more protein than regular yogurt, and its plentiful probiotics make it especially helpful in eliminating waste from the body, which can greatly benefit skin health. Greek yogurt also tastes great and adds other protective and health-promoting nutrients, such as calcium. When combined with apple cider vinegar, Greek yogurt helps to ensure that the internal structures of skin and hair are maintained and promoted naturally.

Per Serving
Calories: 570 | Fat: 39 g | Protein: 26 g | Sodium: 70 mg
Fiber: 6 g | Carbohydrates: 36 g | Sugar: 27 g

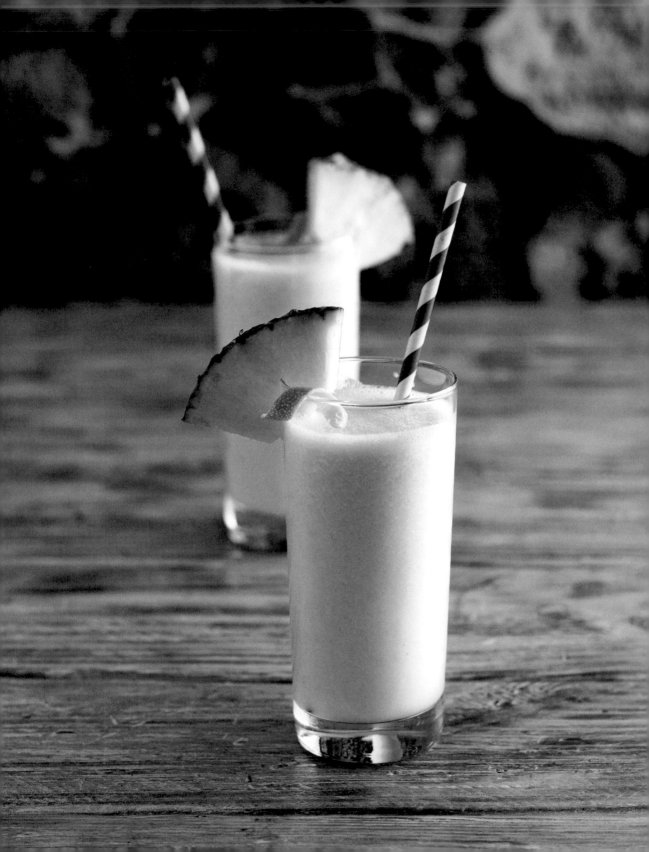

ISLAND TIME

Serves 2

INGREDIENTS

1 tablespoon apple cider vinegar

½ cup aloe vera juice

1 medium banana, peeled and frozen

½ cup chopped pineapple

1 medium orange, peeled and deseeded

2 cups low-fat coconut milk

1 cup ice

---

1 Combine all the ingredients in a large blender.

2 Blend the ingredients on high until thoroughly combined and frothy.

3 Consume immediately or store tightly sealed and refrigerated up to 4 hours.

KEY INGREDIENT: Coconut Milk

While coconut milk is most commonly used in culinary creations like curries, this creamy ingredient is far more versatile than most people think. Coconut milk is packed with nutrients, and its creamy texture improves the quality of drinks like this apple cider vinegar recipe with a richness that can't be matched by any alternative. Coconut milk contains lauric acid, which has been found to have antibacterial, antimicrobial, and antiviral properties. As a result, coconut milk can help boost your immune system and fight diseases that could compromise your body. In addition, coconut milk's vitamin C and copper slow the aging of skin and improve its elasticity, alleviating wrinkles and giving your skin an overall firmer appearance. When clarifying ACV is combined with nourishing coconut milk, the body gets a cleansing and replenishing experience that helps promote health and well-being. Including this drink in your routine provides benefits to your aesthetic appearance while promoting your overall health naturally too!

Per Serving

Calories: 570 | Fat: 39 g | Protein: 26 g | Sodium: 70 mg
Fiber: 6 g | Carbohydrates: 36 g | Sugar: 27 g

CUCUMBER-KIWI BERRY BLAST

Serves 2

INGREDIENTS

1 tablespoon apple cider vinegar
1 medium cucumber, peeled and
  chopped
1 medium kiwi, peeled
1 cup blueberries
1 cup raspberries
2 cups purified water (pH-balanced)

---

1 Combine all the ingredients in a large blender.

2 Blend the ingredients on high until thoroughly combined and frothy.

3 Consume immediately or store tightly sealed and unrefrigerated up to 4 hours.

KEY INGREDIENT: Cucumber

One of the keys to healthy skin and hair is hydration, and at 96 percent water, it's hard to find a food more hydrating than the cucumber. But that's not all there is to love about cucumbers. With massive amounts of vitamins and nutrients that help to replenish and protect the body's cells, the cucumber can improve unhealthy skin and hair with all-natural healing properties that become more powerful when combined with apple cider vinegar. Ensuring that the body's absorption, processing, and utilization of nutrients remains efficient, ACV boosts the work of the cucumber's beautifying mineral, silica. For anyone who seeks supple skin and voluminous hair, delicious and nutritious drinks such as this recipe can be the all-natural answer. Preventing degradation of the very cells that help strengthen hair and promote elasticity of skin, the sound nutrition that comes from cucumbers makes this drink recipe a winner for health, well-being, and astounding aesthetic benefits!

Per Serving
Calories: 110 | Fat: 1 g | Protein: 2 g | Sodium: 5 mg
Fiber: 8 g | Carbohydrates: 26 g | Sugar: 15 g

SWEET CITRUS-KIWI CREAM

Serves 2

INGREDIENTS

1 tablespoon apple cider vinegar
2 cups low-fat vanilla Greek yogurt
1 medium orange, peeled and deseeded
1 medium cucumber, peeled and chopped
2 medium kiwis, peeled
1 cup ice
2 cups purified water (pH-balanced)

1   Combine all the ingredients in a large blender.

2   Blend the ingredients on high until thoroughly combined and frothy.

3   Consume immediately or store tightly sealed and refrigerated up to 4 hours.

KEY INGREDIENT: Kiwi

The deliciously sweet kiwi pumps up this creamy apple cider vinegar drink with nutrients that promote the health of the hair and skin naturally. Kiwis contain more vitamin C than an equivalent amount of oranges, and vitamin C is an effective nutrient for building strong and healthy hair because it builds collagen stores, which are important for both helping hair to grow and for maintaining its strength. The vitamin C in kiwis also helps boost collagen in the skin and keep wrinkles, dryness, and fine lines at bay. When you add the protein from the yogurt that helps strengthen the cell walls in the skin and the strands of the hair, and the ACV for a clarifying effect with a tangy twist, this nutrient-packed drink becomes a sweet and healthy treat. By whipping up this recipe, anyone can enjoy tropical flavors that invigorate the senses while taking in essential nutrition that helps hair and skin.

Per Serving
Calories: 310 | Fat: 6 g | Protein: 22 g | Sodium: 95 mg
Fiber: 5 g | Carbohydrates: 43 g | Sugar: 36 g

SWEET BEETS AND GREENS

Serves 2

INGREDIENTS

- 1 tablespoon apple cider vinegar
- 1 medium red beet, cooked and peeled
- 1 medium yellow beet, cooked and peeled
- 1 cup spinach leaves
- 1 medium banana, peeled and frozen
- 1 cup ice
- 2 cups purified water (pH-balanced)

1 Combine all the ingredients in a large blender.

2 Blend the ingredients on high until thoroughly combined and frothy.

3 Consume immediately or store tightly sealed and unrefrigerated up to 4 hours.

KEY INGREDIENT: Beets

There is so much to love about beets. From their unique earthy taste to their rich colors, beets make a delicious and beautiful addition to any drink. But there's more to beets than meets the eye. Betalains, the important phytochemicals found in beets that are also responsible for their bright color, have antioxidant and anti-inflammatory qualities that work synergistically throughout the body to maintain optimal overall health. Additionally, beets are loaded with folate, which helps the cells to divide properly—a process that is particularly important to the health of the skin. When combined with the nutrition provided by the enzymes, vitamins, and minerals in apple cider vinegar, beets add a depth of color, flavor, and nutrition that can't be compared to that of any other fruit or vegetable.

Per Serving

Calories: 80 | Fat: 0.5 g | Protein: 2 g | Sodium: 60 mg
Fiber: 4 g | Carbohydrates: 20 g | Sugar: 12 g

Chapter 7

RECIPES FOR ANTI-AGING BENEFITS

Commercials and marketing campaigns that promote wrinkle creams, concealers, under-eye products, and skin-firming potions all try to send you the message that beauty can be bought. The truth, however, is that beauty comes from within. Whether you want to look younger, feel younger, or both, the pursuit of an anti-aging goal should start and end with what nutrients and health-improving additions you provide to your body. With the delicious drinks in this chapter you'll find delectable whole foods that pack essential vitamins, minerals, and antioxidants combined with the powerful potency of apple cider vinegar's enzymes and nutrients. This combo creates a rich bounty of essential nutrition on which your body can thrive. While there may not be a fountain of youth, keeping these ACV-based drinks flowing will help restore your youthful glow and vitality quickly, easily, and naturally!

GREAT GRAPE FIZZ

Serves 2

INGREDIENTS

1 tablespoon apple cider vinegar
2 cups Concord grapes
1 medium banana, peeled and frozen
1 cup plain kombucha
1 cup ice
1 cup seltzer water

1 Combine all the ingredients in a large blender.

2 Blend the ingredients on high until thoroughly combined and frothy.

3 Consume immediately or store tightly sealed and unrefrigerated up to 4 hours.

KEY INGREDIENT: Concord Grapes

You may know Concord grapes as the type of grape commonly used to make grape juice or grape jelly, but they have far more uses beyond those sweet treats—as well as a bounty of nutritional benefits. If anti-aging is your goal, then nutrition should play the largest role. One way that Concord grapes can help with this is through their polyphenols. These phytonutrients not only give Concord grapes their color, but they also act as powerful antioxidants that improve overall health by protecting cells from damage. These antioxidants work in tandem with Concord grapes' other nutrients, like vitamin K, to improve certain brain and body processes that have been shown to decline with age, such as memory. Delicious and nutritious foods like Concord grapes make a clean diet designed for anti-aging deliciously simple.

Per Serving

Calories: 130 | Fat: 0.5 g | Protein: 1 g | Sodium: 10 mg
Fiber: 2 g | Carbohydrates: 33 g | Sugar: 23 g

LEMON-LIME CREAM DREAM

Serves 2

INGREDIENTS

1 tablespoon apple cider vinegar
1 tablespoon honey
1 large lemon, peeled and deseeded
1 large lime, peeled and deseeded
2 cups low-fat vanilla Greek yogurt
1 cup ice

1 Combine all the ingredients in a large blender.

2 Blend the ingredients on high until thoroughly combined and frothy.

3 Consume immediately or store tightly sealed and refrigerated up to 4 hours.

KEY INGREDIENT: Lemons

Lemons are packed with plentiful nutrients that are readily used throughout the brain and body for health promotion and illness prevention. In addition to helping to prevent kidney stones, supporting weight loss, aiding in digestion, and fighting cancerous cell growth, lemons help your body stay strong and nimble. The antioxidants in lemons not only help protect the cells in tissues and organs, but they also promote the functioning of the brain, including everything from hormone production and maintenance to cognitive processes, such as memory. Lemons are also an excellent source of vitamin C, which helps produce collagen in the body. Collagen helps to firm and tone the skin, rejuvenating it and reducing wrinkles and other signs of aging. Helping to ensure that nutritional needs are met, clean fruits like lemons that provide nutrients such as vitamin C can help prolong life while improving your health and vitality.

Per Serving

Calories: 270 | Fat: 6 g | Protein: 21 g | Sodium: 95 mg
Fiber: 2 g | Carbohydrates: 38 g | Sugar: 32 g

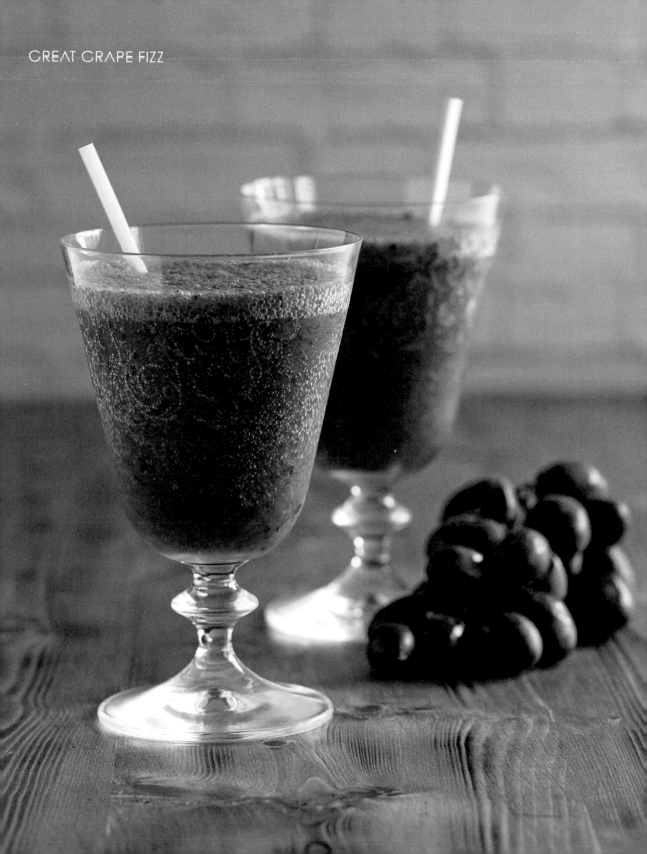

GRAPE GRAPEFRUIT APPLE

Serves 2

INGREDIENTS

1 tablespoon apple cider vinegar
1 cup low-fat plain Greek yogurt
½ cup aloe vera juice
1 medium grapefruit, peeled and
    deseeded
1 large Granny Smith apple, peeled
    and cored
½ cup red seedless grapes
1 cup ice
1 cup purified water (pH-balanced)

---

1 Combine all the ingredients in a large blender.

2 Blend the ingredients on high until thoroughly combined and frothy.

3 Consume immediately or store tightly sealed and refrigerated up to 4 hours.

KEY INGREDIENT: Aloe Vera

If you are concerned with aging, then you should embrace the plentiful benefits of aloe vera as often as possible. Aloe vera contains replenishing nutrients and unique phytochemicals that work to promote proper system functioning throughout the body. Aloe vera helps to protect cells from free radical damage that can lead to serious chronic conditions and diseases. It is also tasteless and odorless, so you can add it to almost any food imaginable. Aloe vera juice contains vitamins A, C, and E among others as well as folic acid and choline. The vitamin A in aloe vera helps maintain healthy vison, bone growth, and immunity; the vitamin C is a powerful immune-boosting vitamin and also builds collagen (which promotes firmer skin and healthy hair); and the vitamin E is a potent antioxidant that prevents cellular damage as you age. Refreshing, replenishing, and nutritious, aloe vera adds anti-aging benefits to apple cider vinegar's already powerful enzymes. To help combat the effects of aging, quality nutrition should be your priority, with foods like aloe vera and ACV being consumed every day.

Per Serving
Calories: 200 | Fat: 3 g | Protein: 13 g | Sodium: 55 mg
Fiber: 4 g | Carbohydrates: 35 g | Sugar: 27 g

WINE NOT?

Serves 2

INGREDIENTS

2 tablespoons apple cider vinegar
1 cup Concord grapes
1 cup green seedless grapes
½ cup green tea prepared with purified water (pH-balanced), cooled
2 cups purified water (pH-balanced)

---

1 Combine all the ingredients in a large blender.

2 Blend the ingredients on high until thoroughly combined and frothy.

3 Consume immediately or store tightly sealed and unrefrigerated up to 4 hours.

KEY INGREDIENT: Green Tea

As you age, the importance of a healthy diet increases. As the brain and body battle the ever-present threats of illness and toxicity in the environment, it is imperative to consume adequate nutrients that help provide protection. Antioxidants like those found in green tea help the cells, tissues, and organs remain free of damage and degradation. In addition, green tea's most abundant polyphenol (antioxidant), EGCG, has been found to reactivate dying skin cells. Called the fountain of youth for skin cells, EGCG caused old skin cells to make DNA and start dividing again. Combining antioxidant-rich green tea with apple cider vinegar increases the nutrients available and adds enzymes that help support anti-aging processes. The vitamins, minerals, antioxidants, and enzymes in this drink all work to promote the healthy functioning of your brain and body. Quick, easy, and nutritious, this drink can be whipped up for a delicious snack that helps to transform the health and healing processes in the body.

Per Serving
Calories: 80 | Fat: 0.5 g | Protein: 1 g | Sodium: 5 mg
Fiber: 1 g | Carbohydrates: 22 g | Sugar: 19 g

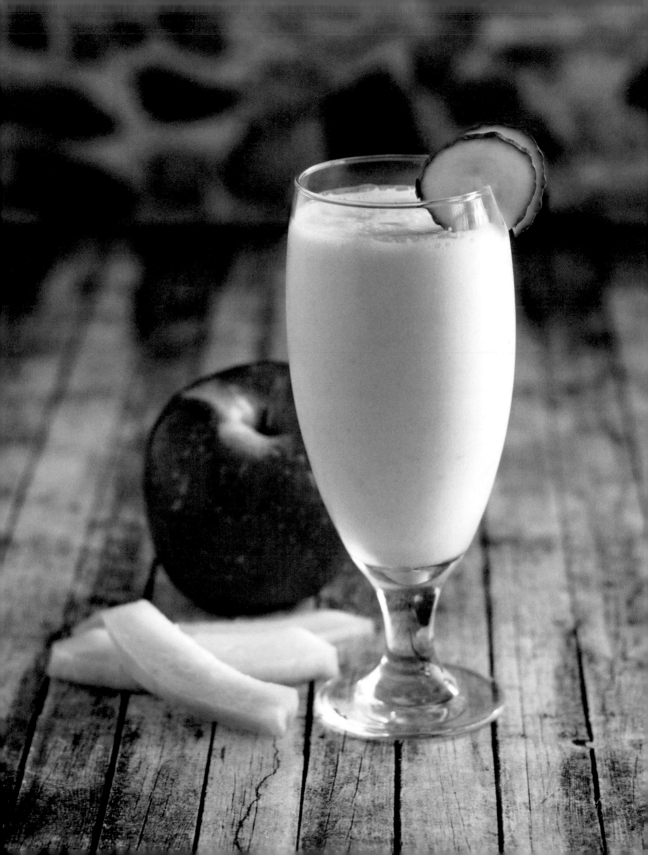

APPLE CUCUMBER HONEYDEW

Serves 2

INGREDIENTS

1 tablespoon apple cider vinegar
1 large Fuji apple, peeled and cored
1 medium cucumber, peeled and chopped
1 cup low-fat vanilla Greek yogurt
1 cup chopped honeydew melon
1 cup ice
1 cup purified water (pH-balanced)

---

1 Combine all the ingredients in a large blender.

2 Blend the ingredients on high until thoroughly combined and frothy.

3 Consume immediately or store tightly sealed and refrigerated up to 4 hours.

KEY INGREDIENT: Honeydew Melon

Packed with vitamins, fiber, and potassium, honeydew melon works to improve the anti-aging health benefits of this delicious apple cider vinegar drink. Honeydew melon contains vitamin C, which is essential to maintaining firmer, younger-looking skin as well as protecting your body from diseases and infections by boosting your immune system. It also contains vitamin B_6, which helps you produce serotonin to regulate your mood and sleep, and potassium, which strengthens your muscles and heart health and reduces high blood pressure. Honeydew melons are also rich in water, making them a hydrating treat for your body. Tantalizing the taste buds and supporting the functions and processes of the body's cells, organs, and systems, this quick and easy treat is the perfect antidote to the effects of aging.

Per Serving
Calories: 210 | Fat: 3 g | Protein: 11 g | Sodium: 65 mg
Fiber: 4 g | Carbohydrates: 36 g | Sugar: 31 g

BLACK AND BLUE BANANAS

Serves 2

INGREDIENTS

1 tablespoon apple cider vinegar
1 cup blackberries
1 cup blueberries
1 medium banana, peeled and
   frozen
2 cups purified water (pH-balanced)

---

1 In a large blender, combine
   the vinegar, blackberries, blueberries, and banana.

2 Blend on high until thoroughly
   combined and frothy.

3 Add the water gradually and
   continue blending until desired
   consistency is reached.

4 Consume immediately or store
   tightly sealed and unrefrigerated up to 4 hours.

KEY INGREDIENT: Blackberries

Rich in all-natural phytochemicals that work as potent anti-oxidants, blackberries help fight damage to the body that comes with aging. When the cells and neurons are protected by effective antioxidants, the incidence of illnesses that are commonly associated with aging can be reduced. In addition to antioxidants, blackberries are also loaded with vitamin C, which can help prevent signs of aging in the skin, such as wrinkles. Manganese—a mineral that is essential for proper brain functioning—is another nutrient that blackberries bring to the table. To top it all off, blackberries are delicious! Sweet and slightly tangy, blackberries improve the flavor and nutrition content of apple cider vinegar drinks like this one, making your anti-aging regimen more enjoyable and effective.

Per Serving
Calories: 130 | Fat: 1 g | Protein: 2 g | Sodium: 4.3 mg
Fiber: 7 g | Carbohydrates: 31 g | Sugar: 18 g

CARROTS AND CREAM

Serves 2

INGREDIENTS

1 tablespoon apple cider vinegar
2 medium carrots, greens removed
1 medium banana
1 cup nonfat vanilla Greek yogurt
1 cup ice
1 cup purified water

1 Combine all the ingredients in a large blender.

2 Blend the ingredients until thoroughly combined and frothy.

3 Consume immediately or store tightly sealed and refrigerated up to 4 hours.

KEY INGREDIENT: Carrots

Carrots add a delicious flavor and vibrant color to any dish or drink, as well as plentiful nutrients that benefit the body and brain. In terms of anti-aging, phytochemicals that are found in natural foods like fruits and vegetables do double duty for promoting health and preventing illness. The body is able to utilize beta-carotene (a phytochemical found in carrots) as a potent antioxidant that helps protect the cells, tissues, and organs from degenerative disease and carcinogenic activity. While protecting the cells from serious chronic illness like cancers, beta-carotene also works to promote the health of the eyes from degenerative conditions such as glaucoma. Combined with ACV's natural enzymes that fight bacterial, viral, and microbial infections that can wreak havoc on the body with age, carrots can be used as an outstanding ingredient in entrées, salads, smoothies, snacks, and drinks (just like this one!) for anti-aging benefits that are simply delicious.

Per Serving
Calories: 170 | Fat: 0.5 g | Protein: 11 g | Sodium: 85 mg
Fiber: 4 g | Carbohydrates: 31 g | Sugar: 21 g

SWEET GREEN PINEAPPLE CREAM

Serves 2

INGREDIENTS

1 tablespoon apple cider vinegar
2 cups low-fat vanilla Greek yogurt
1 cup chopped pineapple
1 medium banana, peeled and
  frozen
1 cup spinach leaves
1 cup ice
½ cup purified water (pH-balanced)

1 In a large blender, combine
  the vinegar, yogurt, pineapple,
  banana, spinach, and ice.

2 Blend on high until thoroughly
  combined and frothy.

3 Add the water gradually and
  continue blending until desired
  consistency is reached.

4 Consume immediately or store
  tightly sealed and refrigerated
  up to 4 hours.

KEY INGREDIENT: Water

The importance of hydration can't be overstated in terms of anti-aging. Adequate water intake is necessary for all of the functions of the body, from maintaining body temperature to removing toxins and wastes, but it's especially important as you get older. Issues that are particularly problematic for aging populations, such as constipation and joint pain, can often be improved simply by drinking more water. In this apple cider vinegar drink, water adds essential hydration while helping to create a smooth, drinkable texture. Quick and easy, this nutritious and delicious drink can make anyone feel younger and revitalized…all thanks to adequate hydration.

Per Serving
Calories: 310 | Fat: 6 g | Protein: 21 g | Sodium: 105 mg
Fiber: 3 g | Carbohydrates: 46 g | Sugar: 37 g

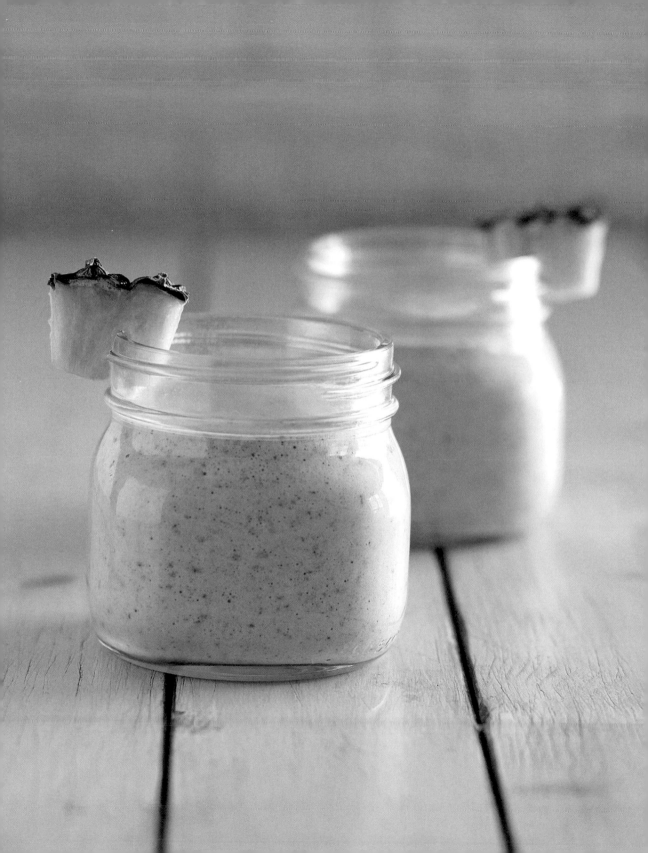

Chapter 8
RECIPES FOR INCREASED IMMUNITY

The quality of your immune system should always be a priority. While moving through an average day, you come into contact with countless bacteria, viruses, microbes, and toxins that can wreak havoc on your immune system. When this constant barrage of environmental and physiological assailants weakens the immune system, the physical results can range from a lack of energy or a simple stuffy nose to far more serious conditions, such as chronic illness. By maintaining a healthy immune system, you can ensure that your body's cells, organs, and systems remain functional and strong. With a special focus on the gut, where between 70 and 80 percent of the immune system's tissue is located, apple cider vinegar's assistance in fighting harmful bacteria and promoting probiotic health greatly benefits the immune system. In addition, the enzymes and nutrients in apple cider vinegar help protect against microbes, bacteria, and viruses. By adding nutrient-dense fruits, vegetables, and other culinary additions to ACV, you can create immunity-boosting smoothies, tonics, and drinks that make staying healthy an enjoyable endeavor!

CREAMY DREAMY VITAMIN C

Serves 2

INGREDIENTS

- 1 tablespoon apple cider vinegar
- 1 medium orange, peeled and deseeded
- 1 cup hulled strawberries
- 1 cup blueberries
- ½ cup chopped pineapple
- 1 cup ice
- 2 cups low-fat vanilla Greek yogurt

1 Combine all the ingredients in a large blender.

2 Blend the ingredients on high until thoroughly combined and frothy.

3 Consume immediately or store tightly sealed and refrigerated up to 4 hours.

KEY INGREDIENT: Strawberries

During their harvest season, strawberries can be purchased fresh from almost any grocer or market. During the off-season, flash-frozen varieties can be purchased, providing the same nutrition content as the fresh berries. Sweet and delicious, strawberries are rich in essential nutrients such as vitamin C, potassium, folic acid, and fiber. In fact, just one cup of strawberries gives you your entire daily requirement of vitamin C, the vitamin that is pivotal to boosting your immunity as well as working as an antioxidant. Quick and easy, this recipe can be consumed as a snack or dessert at any time of the day, making this drink a nutritious option for families, young kids, and people who are on the go. Sipping this delightful drink can be a healthy and pleasurable palate experience year-round!

Per Serving
Calories: 330 | Fat: 6 g | Protein: 22 g | Sodium: 95 mg
Fiber: 5 g | Carbohydrates: 51 g | Sugar: 42 g

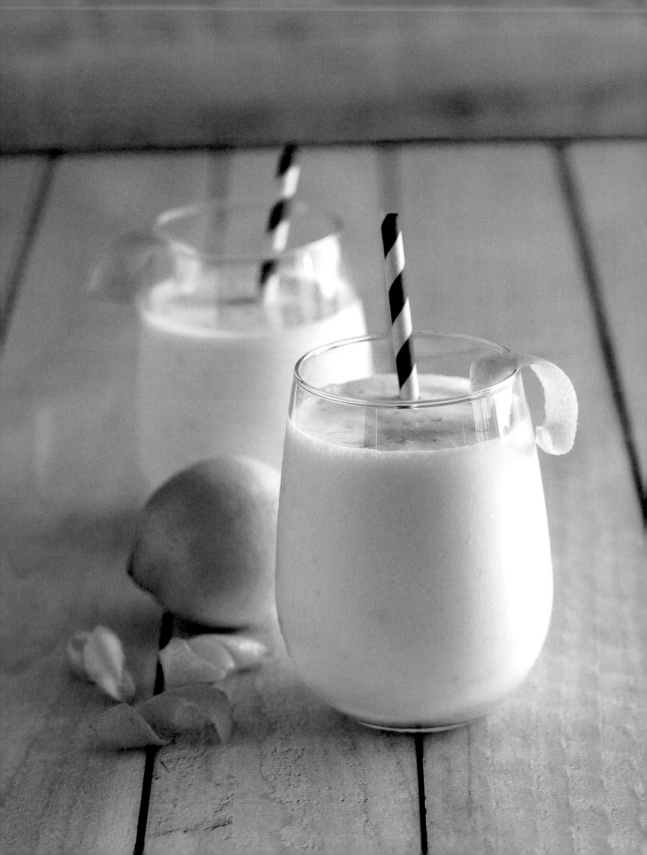

LOTS OF LEMON

Serves 2

INGREDIENTS

1 tablespoon apple cider vinegar
2 cups low-fat vanilla Greek yogurt
3 medium lemons, peeled and
    deseeded
1 teaspoon honey
1 cup ice

---

1 Combine all the ingredients in a large blender.

2 Blend the ingredients on high until thoroughly combined and frothy.

3 Consume immediately or store tightly sealed and refrigerated up to 4 hours.

KEY INGREDIENT: Lemons

Known for their high amounts of vitamin C, lemons make a nutritious addition to your apple cider vinegar drinks any time of year, and especially during the notorious flu season. Helping to support the immune system's functioning, the lemon's vitamins, minerals, and potent antioxidants can also soothe sore throats, calm respiratory illnesses, and fend off viruses, bacterial infections, and microbes that can wreak havoc on the body. When combined with ACV's naturally occurring enzymes, collectively known as "the mother," lemons and other immunity-boosting ingredients can be blended into a delicious and nutritious drink that protects cells and promotes overall health and well-being. When taken at the first sign of symptoms, such as a stuffy nose, a sore throat, or fatigue, this simple drink can help you avoid developing a serious immune system–draining illness.

Per Serving
Calories: 250 | Fat: 6 g | Protein: 21 g | Sodium: 95 mg
Fiber: 2 g | Carbohydrates: 33 g | Sugar: 27 g

SPICY CITRUS-BERRY BLAST

Serves 2

INGREDIENTS

1 tablespoon apple cider vinegar
1 cup chopped pineapple
1 cup blackberries
2 cups low-fat vanilla Greek yogurt
1 tablespoon peeled and grated
  fresh gingerroot
1 cup ice

1 Combine all the ingredients in a large blender.

2 Blend the ingredients on high until thoroughly combined and frothy.

3 Consume immediately or store tightly sealed and refrigerated up to 4 hours.

KEY INGREDIENT: Pineapple

Pineapple is a vitamin C–rich fruit that adds a unique taste to any apple cider vinegar drink. Combined with delicious ingredients like blackberries, yogurt, and ginger, the rich antioxidants in pineapple get a healthy boost that helps to fortify the immune system. The combination of the sweet fruits, the slightly tangy ACV, and the spicy ginger makes for a craving-satisfying combination that ensures that the cells, organs, and systems are provided with ample amounts of the nutrients they need to promote a strong immune system.

Per Serving
Calories: 290 | Fat: 6 g | Protein: 21 g | Sodium: 95 mg
Fiber: 5 g | Carbohydrates: 39 g | Sugar: 33 g

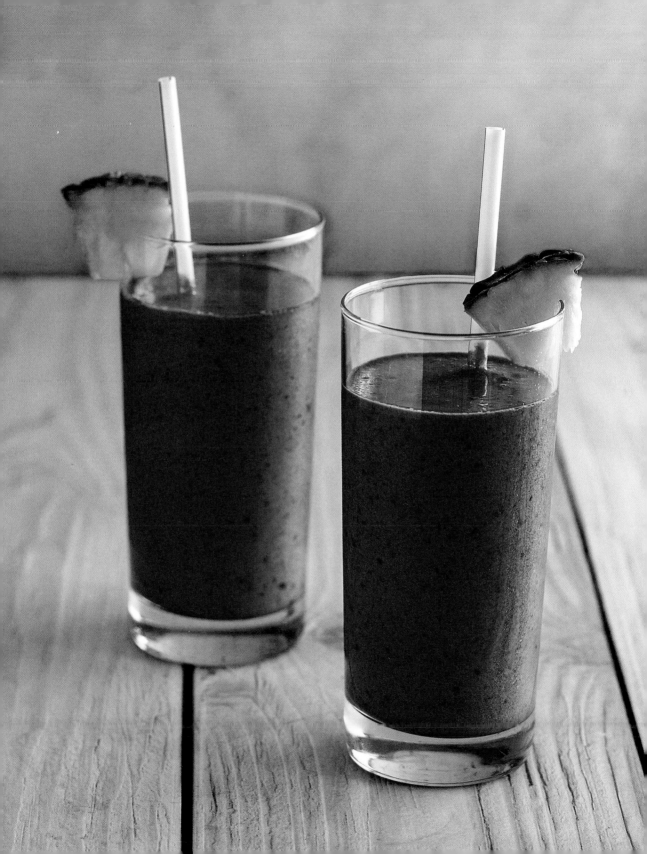

ORANGE-BERRY CREAM

Serves 2

INGREDIENTS

1 tablespoon apple cider vinegar

2 medium oranges, peeled and deseeded

1 cup hulled strawberries

1 cup blueberries

1 cup ice

2 cups low-fat vanilla Greek yogurt

½ cup purified water (pH-balanced)

---

1 In a large blender, combine the vinegar, oranges, strawberries, blueberries, ice, and yogurt.

2 Blend the ingredients on high until thoroughly combined and frothy.

3 Add the water gradually and continue blending until desired consistency is reached.

4 Consume immediately or store tightly sealed and refrigerated up to 4 hours.

KEY INGREDIENT: Oranges

Sweet and slightly tart, fresh oranges add a depth of flavor to this tropical treat that can't be beat by the commercial juice alternatives. Combined with antioxidant-rich berries and the enzymes in apple cider vinegar, these vitamin C–packed oranges help your body stay happy and healthy. Because your body cannot make vitamin C, it's essential to get it from the foods you eat. Vitamin C is necessary for protecting the body's cells, organs, and systems from illness. Vitamin C from natural sources also acts to protect the cells from degradation due to free radical damage. Oranges are not just a sweet treat; they are also the body's best ally in fending off everything from colds and flus to chronic conditions. Adored by even the pickiest of people, the sweet and creamy ingredients in this ACV drink make for the perfect immunity-supporting recipe that can become a staple in your day.

Per Serving

Calories: 340 | Fat: 6 g | Protein: 22 g | Sodium: 95 mg
Fiber: 6 g | Carbohydrates: 53 g | Sugar: 45 g

GINGER-TURMERIC FIZZY TEA WITH ACV

Serves 2

INGREDIENTS

1 tablespoon apple cider vinegar

1 tablespoon peeled and grated fresh gingerroot

1 tablespoon peeled and grated fresh turmeric root

1 teaspoon honey

½ cup plain kombucha

1½ cups black tea prepared with purified water (pH-balanced), cooled

1 In a large blender, combine the vinegar, ginger, turmeric, honey, and kombucha.

2 Blend the ingredients on high until thoroughly combined and frothy.

3 Add the tea gradually and continue blending until desired consistency is reached.

4 Consume immediately or store tightly sealed and unrefrigerated up to 4 hours.

KEY INGREDIENT: Turmeric

With earthy tones and an unexpected depth of flavor, turmeric helps to balance the tang of the kombucha in this apple cider vinegar drink. With acids, enzymes, and antioxidants that all work to support the health of the blood, cells, organs, and tissues, turmeric combines with ACV to prevent the onset of illness naturally. By supporting the body's immune system processes that take place in the gut, turmeric helps to maintain a healthy balance of hormones and enzymes that all work to cleanse the body of "bugs" like bacteria, viruses, and microbes. The all-natural ingredients in this ACV recipe provide the essential nutrients needed for proper immune system functioning. With its woodsy flavor and protective nutrients, turmeric is a simple addition to your drinks that can be an easy way to protect health with every delightful sip!

Per Serving
Calories: 26 | Fat: 0 g | Protein: 0 g | Sodium: 10 mg
Fiber: 0 g | Carbohydrates: 6 g | Sugar: 4 g

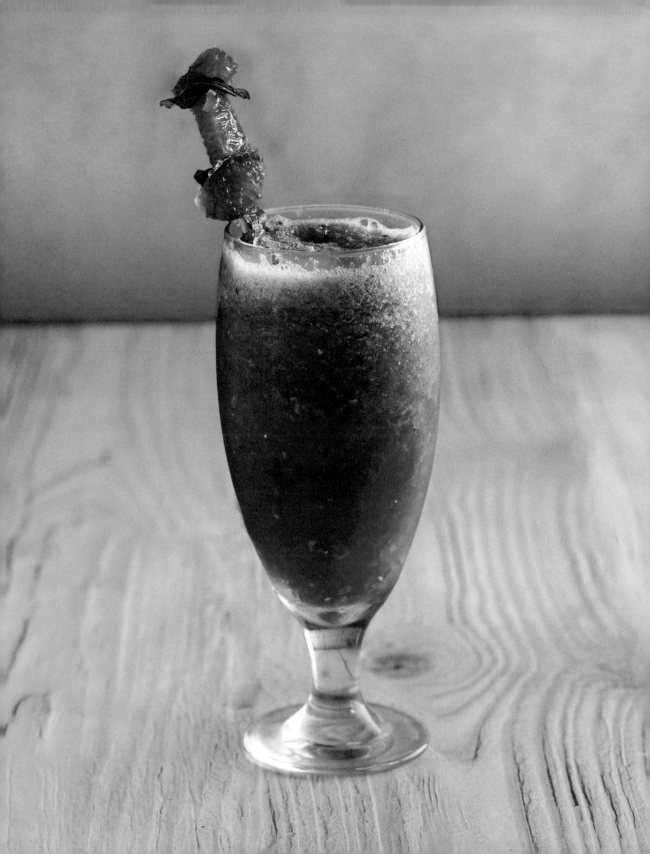

GINGER MINT GRAPEFRUIT

Serves 2

INGREDIENTS

- 1 tablespoon apple cider vinegar
- 2 medium grapefruits, peeled and deseeded
- 1 tablespoon peeled and grated fresh gingerroot
- 1 tablespoon minced fresh mint leaves
- 1 cup ice
- 2 cups white tea prepared with purified water (pH-balanced), cooled

1 In a large blender, combine the vinegar, grapefruits, ginger, mint, and ice.

2 Blend the ingredients on high until thoroughly combined and frothy.

3 Add the tea gradually and continue blending until desired consistency is reached.

4 Consume immediately or store tightly sealed and unrefrigerated up to 4 hours.

KEY INGREDIENT: Ginger

Ginger provides the body with protection and preservation of the immune system while adding slightly sweet and spicy flavors to any recipe. Its power comes from gingerols, chemical compounds that have astounding antioxidant and anti-inflammatory qualities. Ginger and apple cider vinegar combine to create the perfect drink for immunity due to their enzymes and antioxidants that specifically promote gut health. The gut is where most of the immune system's work is done, protecting the body from infection by purging impurities, toxins, and microbes that could be harmful to overall health. By supporting the metabolic processes and organ functioning that lead to strong immunity, ginger and ACV work to protect the body from the inside out. Adding this delightfully spicy root to your favorite ACV drink makes for a delicious and nutritious treat that can be made easily and quickly.

Per Serving

Calories: 90 | Fat: 0.5 g | Protein: 2 g | Sodium: 15 mg
Fiber: 3 g | Carbohydrates: 21 g | Sugar: 18 g

SPICY GREENS AND CUCUMBERS WITH ACV

Serves 2

INGREDIENTS

- 1 tablespoon apple cider vinegar
- 1 tablespoon peeled and grated fresh gingerroot
- 2 medium cucumbers, peeled and chopped
- 1 cup chopped kale leaves, ribs removed
- 2 cups purified water (pH-balanced)

1 In a large blender, combine the vinegar, ginger, cucumbers, and kale.

2 Blend the ingredients on high until thoroughly combined and frothy.

3 Add the water gradually and continue blending until desired consistency is reached.

4 Consume immediately or store tightly sealed and unrefrigerated up to 4 hours.

KEY INGREDIENT: Kale

Some people find the leaves of kale a bit too bitter for their taste, but the benefits for the immune system that kale provides are too plentiful to disregard this leafy green. With astounding amounts of vitamin C, vitamin K, and phytochemicals that do double duty as antioxidants, kale provides protection to the body's cells that improve immunity. Luckily, the other ingredients in this apple cider vinegar drink recipe help mask the flavor of the deep-green vegetable and combat any bitterness. The ACV in this recipe helps with the absorption and utilization of the nutrients provided by the other ingredients, ensuring that the immune system gets the nutrition it needs. Including kale in your daily diet is no longer a chore when you add this delicious ACV drink to your routine.

Per Serving

Calories: 60 | Fat: 1 g | Protein: 3 g | Sodium: 20 mg
Fiber: 3 g | Carbohydrates: 14 g | Sugar: 6 g

SALAD SMOOTHIE

Serves 2

INGREDIENTS

- 1 tablespoon apple cider vinegar
- 1 cup chopped romaine leaves, ribs removed
- 1 cup chopped kale leaves, ribs removed
- 1 medium tomato, chopped
- 1 tablespoon oregano oil
- 2 cups purified water (pH-balanced)

1. In a large blender, combine the vinegar, romaine, kale, tomato, and oregano oil.

2. Blend the ingredients on high until thoroughly combined and frothy.

3. Add the water gradually and continue blending until desired consistency is reached.

4. Consume immediately or store tightly sealed and unrefrigerated up to 4 hours.

KEY INGREDIENT: Oregano Oil

Greens and other salad staples are being included in smoothies and drinks more and more. Rather than opting for the commercially made drinks that contain common salad ingredients, creating your own at-home versions, like this delicious recipe, can promote health without the unwanted ingredients and additives used as preservatives in store-bought alternatives. Oregano oil is an outstanding ingredient that can be added to your favorite savory recipes, helping to protect the respiratory system, promote immune system functions, and support cell and organ health throughout the body. With a growing percentage of the population becoming more aware of the natural protective properties in oregano oil, this once-rare ingredient is becoming more popular and easy to find. If you love oregano's taste, you'll fall in love with oregano oil and start finding new, exciting ways to include it in your daily diet.

Per Serving
Calories: 90 | Fat: 7 g | Protein: 2 g | Sodium: 20 mg
Fiber: 2 g | Carbohydrates: 6 g | Sugar: 3 g

Chapter 9

RECIPES FOR INCREASED ENERGY

Energy is required for every function performed by the body. In addition to the energy you need to go for a jog, wash your car, or run your daily errands, your body's systems require energy to perform functions such as allowing your heart to beat, your brain to process thoughts, and your stomach to digest food. It takes massive amounts of energy to perform physiological functions and daily activities, so a lack of energy can be catastrophic. In order to maintain the levels of energy needed to enjoy everyday life healthfully and happily, look no further than your trusted bottle of apple cider vinegar! With nutrients and enzymes that support the body's functions that produce and promote energy, ACV encourages all of the body's networks to work synergistically to maximize energy levels throughout the day. The drinks and smoothies in this chapter will help you combine vibrant fruits, vegetables, and other culinary treats with ACV for a naturally nutritious and delicious approach to energizing your body and mind.

WACKY WATERMELON WONDER

Serves 2

INGREDIENTS

- 1 tablespoon apple cider vinegar
- 1 tablespoon peeled and grated fresh gingerroot
- 4 cups chopped watermelon, deseeded
- ½ cup plain kombucha

1 Combine all the ingredients in a large blender.

2 Blend the ingredients on high until thoroughly combined and frothy.

3 Consume immediately or store tightly sealed and unrefrigerated up to 4 hours.

KEY INGREDIENT: Kombucha

Kombucha is an ancient beverage made by fermenting sweetened tea. Kombucha adds countless phytochemicals, antioxidants, and enzymes that all work to support metabolism—the process primarily responsible for promoting energy levels. The nutrient-dense ingredients in this apple cider vinegar drink make pumping up your energy a deliciously easy task. The kombucha in this recipe not only helps to protect cells, improve immunity, and maximize metabolism, but it also helps to cleanse the bloodstream and gut of impurities and toxins that can interfere with energy and focus. Delicious and nutritious, kombucha's unique flavors come with energy benefits that can't be beat.

Per Serving
Calories: 100 | Fat: 0.5 g | Protein: 2 g | Sodium: 10 mg
Fiber: 1 g | Carbohydrates: 25 g | Sugar: 19 g

SPICY GINGER TEA WITH ACV

Serves 4

INGREDIENTS

- 2 tablespoons apple cider vinegar
- 1 (1") piece gingerroot, peeled and sliced
- 1 tablespoon honey
- 2 cups green tea prepared with purified water (pH-balanced), cooled

1 Add all the ingredients to a large pitcher.

2 Stir until all the ingredients are thoroughly combined.

3 Cover and refrigerate 2–4 hours. Keep tea stored in refrigerator up to 24 hours.

KEY INGREDIENT: Green Tea

In addition to offering ample amounts of protective antioxidants, green tea also helps to improve energy production with natural stores of caffeine. Acting to support the body's processing of nutrients, green tea's phytochemicals, such as catechins, protect the cells against harmful degradation. Also protecting the hormonal balance in the body and brain, green tea's nutrients and phytochemicals ensure that the very sources responsible for metabolic processes and "feel-good" hormone production remain functioning as intended. Apple cider vinegar drinks like this one can be made quickly and easily and consumed at home or on the go. Whether the reason for the energy depletion is illness or simply fatigue, green tea's combination with ACV makes for a simple (and delicious) solution.

Per Serving
Calories: 18 | Fat: 0 g | Protein: 0 g | Sodium: 1.5 mg
Fiber: 0 g | Carbohydrates: 5 g | Sugar: 4 g

SWEET BEET TREAT

Serves 2

INGREDIENTS

1 tablespoon apple cider vinegar

1 medium red beet, roasted and peeled

1 medium yellow beet, roasted and peeled

1 medium Granny Smith apple, peeled and cored

1 cup ice

2 cups purified water (pH-balanced)

1 Combine all the ingredients in a large blender.

2 Blend the ingredients on high until thoroughly combined and frothy.

3 Consume immediately or store tightly sealed and unrefrigerated up to 4 hours.

KEY INGREDIENT: Beets

With phytochemicals that promote the overall health and wellness of the body's cells, organs, and systems, beets support the production of energy by maintaining important metabolic processes. Regulating hormones, maintaining proper hydration, and maximizing the absorption, utilization, and distribution of essential nutrients, sweet beets are a delicious addition to any diet designed for sustained energy. Beets provide plentiful phytochemicals and nutrients such as B vitamins, iron, manganese, copper, magnesium, and potassium that all work together in maintaining energy levels for hours. Beets have also been shown to improve your stamina and endurance. In studies involving athletes, the nitrates in beets helped boost their endurance performance, allowing them to keep active longer than participants who didn't consume beets. With a colorful variety of beets becoming more readily available year-round throughout the country, you can whip up an ACV drink recipe containing sweet beets for an instantaneous boost in energy.

Per Serving
Calories: 70 | Fat: 0 g | Protein: 1 g | Sodium: 50 mg
Fiber: 4 g | Carbohydrates: 16 g | Sugar: 11 g

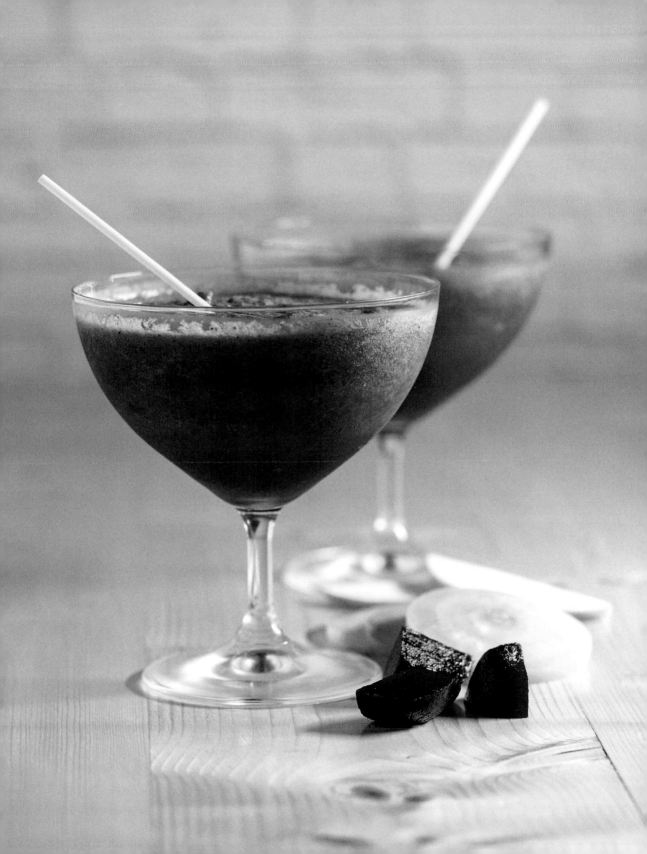

MELON MADNESS

Serves 2

INGREDIENTS

1 tablespoon apple cider vinegar

1 cup chopped watermelon, deseeded

1 cup chopped cantaloupe

1 cup chopped honeydew melon

1½ cups low-fat vanilla Greek yogurt

½ cup plain kombucha

1 cup ice

½ cup purified water (pH-balanced)

---

1 Combine the vinegar, watermelon, cantaloupe, honeydew, yogurt, kombucha, and ice in a large blender.

2 Blend the ingredients on high until thoroughly combined and frothy.

3 Add the water gradually and continue blending until desired consistency is reached.

4 Consume immediately or store tightly sealed and refrigerated up to 4 hours.

KEY INGREDIENT: Watermelon

Anyone struggling with energy-related conditions like chronic fatigue, cognitive challenges, or difficulties staying active can benefit from the inclusion of nutrient-dense foods in their daily diet. Containing easily absorbable moisture and essential nutrients like vitamin C and lycopene, watermelon adds a sweet flavor and the energy-supporting dietary elements your body requires. Lycopene is not only the phytonutrient that gives watermelon its red color; it's also an incredible antioxidant with pain-fighting, cancer-preventing, and brain-boosting powers. Sweet fruits like cantaloupe and watermelon, along with creamy ingredients like yogurt, maximize the flavor sensations and nutrition content of this apple cider vinegar drink.

Per Serving

Calories: 250 | Fat: 5 g | Protein: 16 g | Sodium: 100 mg
Fiber: 2 g | Carbohydrates: 38 g | Sugar: 35 g

CHAI TEA WITH ACV

Serves 2

INGREDIENTS

- 1 tablespoon apple cider vinegar
- 1 tablespoon ground cardamom
- 1 teaspoon ground cloves
- 1 cup ice
- 1 cup white tea prepared with purified water (pH-balanced), cooled
- 1 cup unsweetened vanilla almond milk
- 1 tablespoon honey

1 Combine all the ingredients in a large blender.

2 Blend the ingredients on high until thoroughly combined and frothy.

3 Consume immediately or store tightly sealed and refrigerated up to 4 hours.

KEY INGREDIENT: Cardamom

Spices are normally added to dishes and drinks for their fantastic flavors and invigorating aromas, but they are also nutritional powerhouses. Cardamom is one such spice that is well known for its inclusion in certain dishes and drinks like chai tea. While commercial chai teas are popular, many of these prepared options contain unhealthy ingredients, excessive amounts of sugar, and harsh additives and preservatives that all contribute to a depletion of energy. At-home creations like this apple cider vinegar drink provide astounding amounts of nutrients that all work to promote energy and avoid the inevitable "crash" that follows blood sugar spikes. Along with the benefit of improved energy, spices like cardamom add a dose of protective and preventative phytochemicals that also work to improve immunity. Delicious, nutritious, and loaded with essential enzymes, this drink recipe is one of the most delightful ways to boost your energy naturally.

Per Serving
Calories: 70 | Fat: 2 g | Protein: 1 g | Sodium: 95 mg
Fiber: 2 g | Carbohydrates: 13 g | Sugar: 9 g

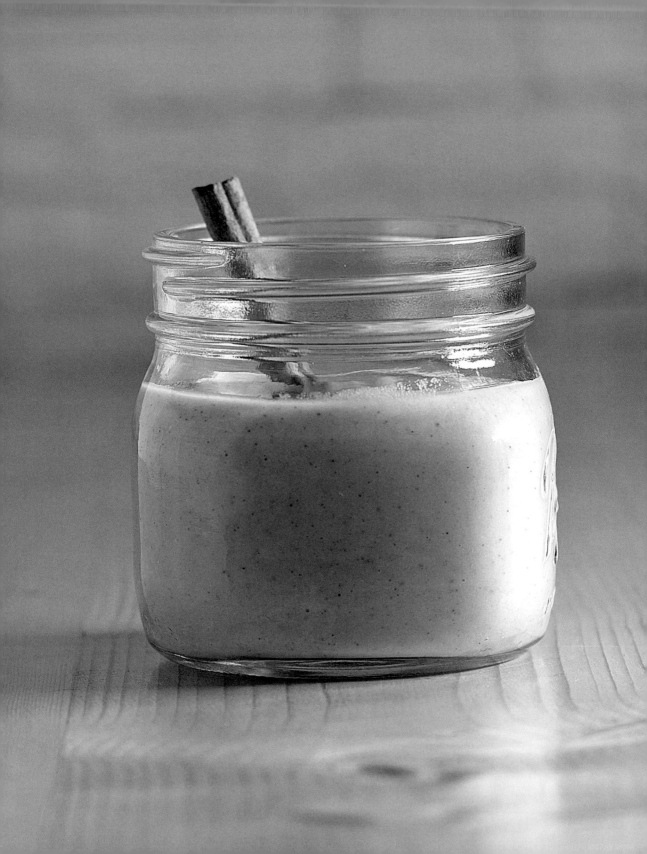

CREAMY SWEET POTATO PIE

Serves 2

INGREDIENTS

- 1 tablespoon apple cider vinegar
- 1 teaspoon ground cinnamon
- 1 teaspoon ground ginger
- 1 teaspoon ground cloves
- 1 large sweet potato, cooked and peeled
- 1 cup low-fat plain Greek yogurt
- 1 cup unsweetened vanilla almond milk
- 1 cup ice

1 Combine all the ingredients in a large blender.

2 Blend the ingredients on high until thoroughly combined and frothy.

3 Consume immediately or store tightly sealed and refrigerated up to 4 hours.

KEY INGREDIENT: Sweet Potatoes

Complex carbohydrates like those found in sweet potatoes are ideal for steady supplies of energy. Because they release glucose into your system more gradually than other foods, they reduce the sugar high/crash cycle and keep you going strong all day long. In addition, sweet potatoes are high in vitamin C, beta-carotene, magnesium, and iron—all of which are essential energy boosters. This apple cider vinegar drink recipe uses sweet potatoes as its star ingredient, with plentiful nutrients that can be utilized in every step of the body's energy-production processes. Combining sweet potatoes with protein-rich yogurt and nutrient-dense spices, like cinnamon, leads to a tasty drink that increases energy naturally. Quick and easy to create, this sweet recipe makes clean drinking for energy the best part of any busy day.

Per Serving
Calories: 190 | Fat: 4 g | Protein: 14 g | Sodium: 170 mg Fiber: 5 g | Carbohydrates: 26 g | Sugar: 10 g

SWEET RED LEMONY LIFT

Serves 2

INGREDIENTS

1 tablespoon apple cider vinegar

2 cups hulled strawberries

2 medium lemons, peeled and deseeded

1 tablespoon honey

1 cup ice

2 cups purified water (pH-balanced)

---

1 In a large blender, combine the vinegar, strawberries, lemons, honey, and ice.

2 Blend the ingredients on high until thoroughly combined and frothy.

3 Add the water gradually and continue blending until desired consistency is reached.

4 Consume immediately or store tightly sealed and unrefrigerated up to 4 hours.

KEY INGREDIENT: Honey

With a unique sweetness, honey adds an exceptional taste sensation to all sorts of dishes and drinks. One of the most impressive aspects of honey is how its phytochemicals and nutrients provide outstanding support to the body's metabolism and energy production. Helping to prevent illnesses produced by bacterial, viral, and microbial infections, the addition of honey increases the protective properties provided by other nutrient-dense ingredients in this recipe. With a lower glycemic index rating than both white and brown sugar, honey makes a sweet addition to apple cider vinegar drinks like this one without worry about blood sugar spikes. If you find that energy issues plague your day, try out this delicious and nutritious ACV drink for energy that lasts for hours.

Per Serving

Calories: 100 | Fat: 1 g | Protein: 2 g | Sodium: 5 mg
Fiber: 5 g | Carbohydrates: 25 g | Sugar: 17 g

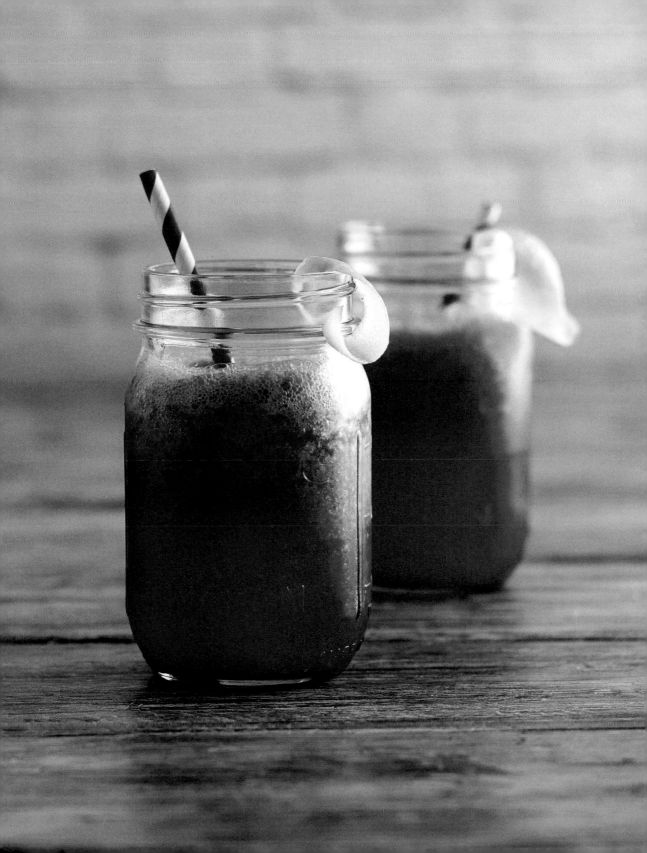

BERRY "FRO-YO"

Serves 2

INGREDIENTS

1 tablespoon apple cider vinegar
1 cup raspberries
1 cup hulled strawberries
1 cup blackberries
1 medium banana, peeled
2 cups low-fat plain frozen yogurt
1 cup ice

1 Combine all the ingredients in a large blender.

2 Blend the ingredients on high until thoroughly combined and desired thickness is reached.

3 Consume immediately or store tightly sealed and in a freezer up to 72 hours.

KEY INGREDIENT: Strawberries

Strawberries have several energy-boosting capabilities. Strawberries contain natural sugars, which give you an energy boost, as well as vitamin C and fiber, which will keep you alert and functioning throughout the day. There is also new research that shows that strawberries can boost cognitive functioning, helping to keep you more alert and focused. Making almost any dish into a nutritious treat, strawberries can also be added to apple cider vinegar drinks like this delightful recipe to create a sweet treat that makes eating for energy an easy pursuit. With the combination of healthy and delicious ingredients in this drink, all aspects of the body can work synergistically to maintain cell health, improve immunity, and protect the organs and systems from complications that can jeopardize energy levels. This recipe promotes cognitive processes and maintains your overall health, thereby helping you to sustain energy levels in a tasty and nutritious way.

Per Serving
Calories: 329 | Fat: 4.5 g | Protein: 13 g | Sodium: 65 mg
Fiber: 11 g | Carbohydrates: 61 g | Sugar: 44 g

Chapter 10

RECIPES FOR REDUCING INFLAMMATION

Inflammation is the body's natural response to injury or illness. By flooding the affected area with helpful blood cells and reparative biochemicals, the body can repair wounds, ward off infection, and heal painful breaks and bruises. When inflammation progresses from an acute response to an isolated incident into a chronic state, serious health conditions can result. Over time, chronic inflammation can contribute to debilitating health issues, such as arthritis, cellular changes such as those seen in cancer, and hormonal imbalances that plague the body with the threat of diseases that would otherwise be avoided. Luckily, you can combat inflammation naturally with a clean diet low in or free of sodium, sugar, unhealthy fats, and additives, along with a daily regimen that includes apple cider vinegar. The drink recipes in this chapter will help you strike back at inflammation by whipping up sweet smoothies and savory drinks that calm the affected area and speed recovery. While drinking your anti-inflammatory, ACV-based concoctions, you can enjoy the added benefits of improved mobility, increased energy, and maximized metabolic functioning, all of which help to get the body moving again.

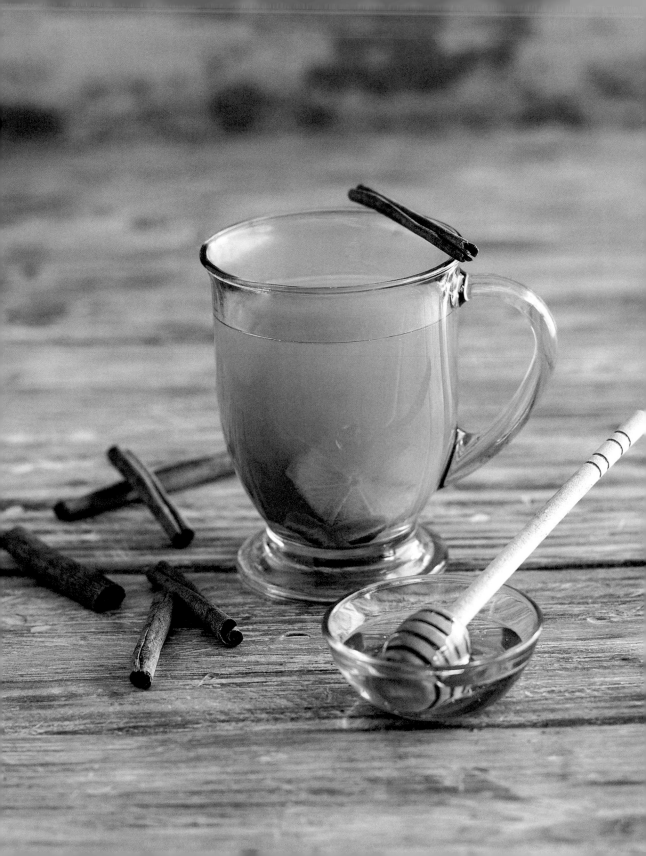

TURMERIC TODDY

Serves 2

INGREDIENTS

1 teaspoon ground turmeric
½ teaspoon ground cloves
1 teaspoon ground cinnamon
1 tablespoon honey
2 cups hot purified water (pH-
   balanced)
1 tablespoon apple cider vinegar
1 medium lemon, peeled, deseeded,
   and sliced

---

1 In a shaker, combine turmeric,
   cloves, cinnamon, honey, and
   hot water.

2 Shake vigorously until thoroughly combined and frothy.

3 Add vinegar and lemon, and
   allow to steep 5–10 minutes.

4 Consume immediately or store
   tightly sealed and unrefrigerated up to 4 hours.

KEY INGREDIENT: Turmeric

The most commonly consumed version of the hot toddy is packed with alcohol and includes unhealthy sweet additions that are used to even out an otherwise tart flavor. By making your own toddy recipe at home, you can easily swap out unhealthy ingredients for healthy alternatives like turmeric that create the same taste experience but offer increased benefits to the body. Turmeric is a bright yellow spice commonly used in dishes like curries that contains an active ingredient called curcumin. Curcumin is an antioxidant that has anti-inflammatory properties that can reduce swelling (inflammation) and help with conditions such as arthritis, muscle pain and injury, and inflammatory bowel disease among others. Inflammation can wreak havoc on your body's organs, joints, and tissues, giving you bouts of discomfort and even illness that compromise your well-being. Because the incidence of inflammation can be acute or chronic, it is imperative to eat a diet consisting of clean foods that prevent inflammation, such as turmeric and apple cider vinegar. The addition of antimicrobial honey and antioxidant-rich lemons to this drink make fighting inflammation a winning battle.

Per Serving
Calories: 40 | Fat: 0 g | Protein: 0 g | Sodium: 2.3 mg
Fiber: 1 g | Carbohydrates: 11 g | Sugar: 9 g

OH-SO-NICE GINGER SPICE

Serves 2

INGREDIENTS

1 tablespoon apple cider vinegar

1 tablespoon peeled and grated fresh gingerroot

½ teaspoon ground cloves

1 tablespoon honey

1 cup ice

2 cups unsweetened vanilla almond milk

---

1 Combine all the ingredients in a large blender.

2 Blend the ingredients on high until thoroughly combined and frothy.

3 Consume immediately or store tightly sealed and refrigerated up to 4 hours.

KEY INGREDIENT: Ginger

The unique compounds in ginger, gingerols, help to make this delicious apple cider vinegar drink a natural preventative for painful inflammation. With a well-founded concern that chronic inflammation can lead to permanent conditions such as arthritis and even cell mutation, many people are turning to all-natural ingredients like ginger and ACV to promote the body's natural defense against inflammation, regardless of where and when the inflammation occurs. Nutrient-dense ingredients like ginger and ACV can not only prevent the onset of inflammation, but they can also help alleviate symptoms that occur when inflammation sets in. Anyone hoping to treat their inflammation naturally can opt for the delicious taste and aroma of ginger in this drink instead of over-the-counter and prescription alternatives.

Per Serving
Calories: 80 | Fat: 3.5 g | Protein: 1 g | Sodium: 190 mg
Fiber: 1 g | Carbohydrates: 11 g | Sugar: 9 g

GARLICKY GREEN TOMATO-BASIL

Serves 2

INGREDIENTS

1 tablespoon apple cider vinegar

1 cup spinach leaves

1 large kale leaf with ribs removed, chopped

2 large tomatoes, chopped

1 clove garlic, peeled

½ cup whole basil leaves

½ medium avocado, peeled and pitted

2 cups purified water (pH-balanced)

---

1 Combine all the ingredients in a large blender.

2 Blend the ingredients on high until thoroughly combined and frothy.

3 Consume immediately or store tightly sealed and unrefrigerated up to 4 hours.

KEY INGREDIENT: Garlic

When you're craving a savory selection for fighting inflammation, this delicious apple cider vinegar drink can be the perfect answer. By adding ingredients like garlic—with its inflammation-fighting antioxidant, allicin—the benefits of this drink can be astounding. Rich in anti-inflammatory foods, concoctions like this recipe can leave you feeling satisfied while purging the body, blood, and brain of toxins, inflammatory proteins, and other elements that can contribute to the development of inflammation. By consistently including whole, natural foods, such as those found here, anyone suffering from inflammatory illness can proactively protect his or her entire body against the degradation caused by inflammatory elements. Because early symptoms of inflammation can be easy to miss or be misdiagnosed, including anti-inflammatory foods such as garlic in your diet can help ensure that the body has all it needs to fight inflammation effectively and naturally.

Per Serving

Calories: 110 | Fat: 6 g | Protein: 4 g | Sodium: 35 mg
Fiber: 6 g | Carbohydrates: 14 g | Sugar: 6 g

PINK PINEAPPLE PERFECTION

Serves 2

INGREDIENTS

1 tablespoon apple cider vinegar
2 cups chopped pineapple
1 cup raspberries
1 cup low-fat plain Greek yogurt
1 cup unsweetened vanilla almond
  milk
1 cup ice

1 Combine all the ingredients in
   a large blender.

2 Blend the ingredients on high
   until thoroughly combined and
   frothy.

3 Consume immediately or store
   tightly sealed and refrigerated
   up to 4 hours.

KEY INGREDIENT: Raspberries

Raspberries are a powerhouse of nutrients and vitamins that can help with conditions such as obesity, cancer, and inflammation. The amount and diversity of antioxidants and anti-inflammatory phytonutrients in raspberries is noteworthy, and includes anthocyanins, flavonols, tannins, and ellagic acid. These phytonutrients protect you from oxidative stress and the dangers of excessive inflammation by helping to scavenge free radical molecules and by regulating the enzymes that could trigger unwanted inflammation. In addition, the ellagic acid in raspberries has been shown to prevent overactivity of pro-inflammatory enzymes and to hinder their overproduction. The combination of fruits and natural drinks like apple cider vinegar is extremely effective at fighting inflammation. The natural antioxidants and phytochemicals in these foods are able to work hand in hand with the body's systems to safeguard the cells, organs, tissues, and joints from the conditions that contribute to the development of this debilitating issue. You can prevent inflammation and speed your body's healing safely and naturally by adding raspberries to delicious drinks such as this recipe.

Per Serving
Calories: 210 | Fat: 4 g | Protein: 9 g | Sodium: 180 mg
Fiber: 7 g | Carbohydrates: 37 g | Sugar: 27 g

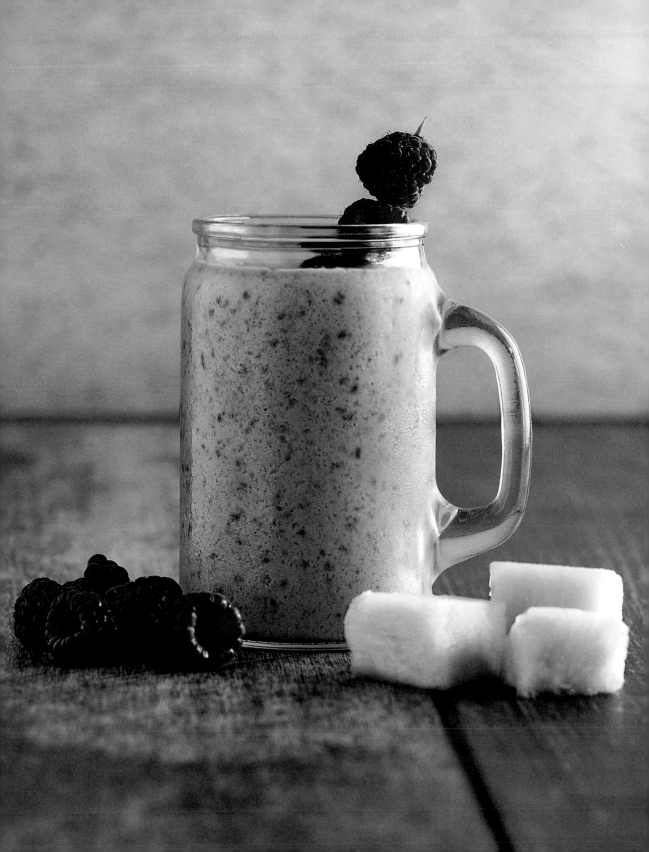

GREAT GRAPE PEAR

Serves 2

INGREDIENTS

1 tablespoon apple cider vinegar
2 cups green seedless grapes
1 medium pear, peeled and cored
2 cups organic apple juice (not from
   concentrate)

1 Combine all the ingredients in
   a large blender.

2 Blend the ingredients on high
   until thoroughly combined and
   frothy.

3 Consume immediately or store
   tightly sealed and unrefrigerated up to 4 hours.

KEY INGREDIENT: Grapes

With anti-inflammatory phytochemicals like resveratrol, grapes can help improve any diet aimed at reducing inflammation naturally. Effectively purging inflammatory proteins that can wreak havoc on the body and brain, clean whole foods like grapes make for a delicious addition to foods, snacks, and drinks. If your goal is improving your overall health with a focus on fighting inflammation, delicious and nutritious foods can make a major difference. While it can be challenging at times to adhere to a clean diet, sweet fruits and crunchy vegetables can combine to provide necessary nutrients while offering up flavors and textures that please the palate. Apple cider vinegar and grapes join forces in this drink to provide the body with all-natural nutrition that prevents the development of inflammation in the body easily and naturally.

Per Serving
Calories: 260 | Fat: 0.5 g | Protein: 2 g | Sodium: 30 mg
Fiber: 4 g | Carbohydrates: 68 g | Sugar: 60 g

PEACH-BERRY CRUMBLE WITH GINGER

Serves 2

INGREDIENTS

1 tablespoon apple cider vinegar
1 cup raspberries
1 cup blueberries
2 medium peaches, pitted
1 tablespoon peeled and grated
   fresh gingerroot
1 cup ice
2 cups low-fat vanilla Greek yogurt
¼ cup low-fat granola

1   Combine all the ingredients in
    a large blender.

2   Blend the ingredients on high
    until thoroughly combined and
    frothy.

3   Consume immediately or store
    tightly sealed and refrigerated
    up to 4 hours.

KEY INGREDIENT: Peaches

Peaches' vibrant coloring is one of the first indicators of their rich stores of nutrients. The phytochemicals in yellow and orange foods are powerful antioxidants that protect against inflammation, making peaches one of the top recommended fruits for anti-inflammatory diets. With a delicious taste and a tantalizing texture, the juice, flesh, and skin of peaches all contribute to the nutritional profile of this apple cider vinegar drink. Other benefits to the body from this nutrient-dense fruit include cleansed blood, improved cognitive functioning, reduced bruising, and maximized nutrient absorption. While the inclusion of peaches in apple cider vinegar drinks is a great step toward reducing inflammation, the addition of the berries and ginger can help ensure that the antioxidants that are absorbed are all helpful in preventing inflammation and improving overall health and wellness.

Per Serving
Calories: 420 | Fat: 10 g | Protein: 24 g | Sodium: 100 mg
Fiber: 9 g | Carbohydrates: 63 g | Sugar: 47 g

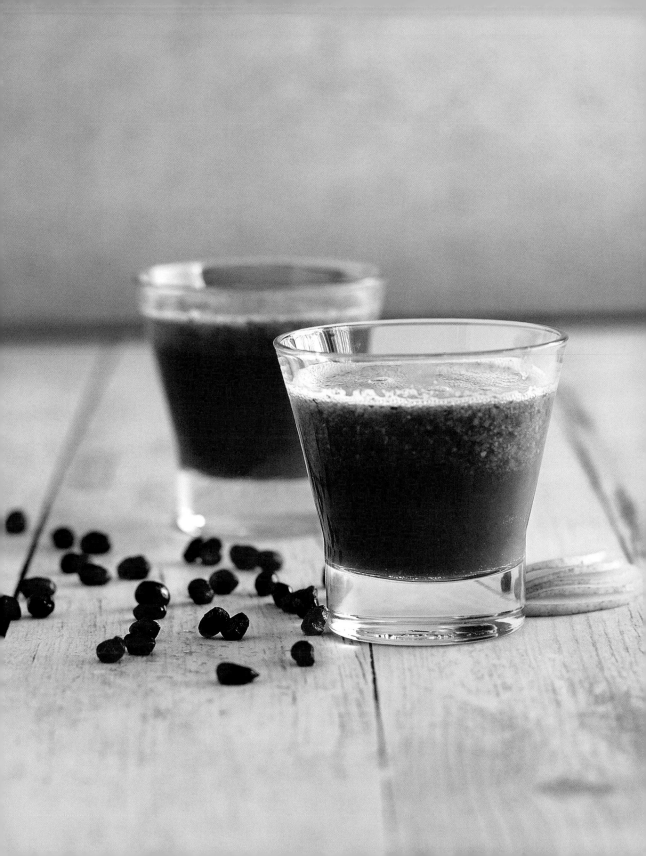

POMEGRANATE-PEAR PAIN RELIEVER

Serves 2

INGREDIENTS

1 tablespoon apple cider vinegar
1 teaspoon honey
1 cup pomegranate arils (jewels)
1 medium pear, peeled and cored
2 cups green tea prepared with puri-
    fied water (pH-balanced), cooled
1 cup ice

1 Combine all the ingredients in
   a large blender.

2 Blend the ingredients on high
   until thoroughly combined and
   frothy.

3 Consume immediately or store
   tightly sealed and unrefrigerated up to 4 hours.

KEY INGREDIENT: Pomegranate

Pomegranates contain fiber, vitamins C and K, folate, and potassium, but their real claim to fame is their levels of antioxidants. In a recent study pomegranates beat blueberry juice, acai juice, and Concord grape juice for antioxidant potency because pomegranates contain the most of *every* type of antioxidant. Pomegranates have shown to work their anti-inflammatory activity in the gut, in tissues, and in the brain. In addition, the antioxidants in pomegranates may also help reduce the inflammation that contributes to the destruction of cartilage in your joints, making it a natural way to reduce joint and arthritis pain and symptoms. Since inflammation can lead to countless dysfunctions in the body, pomegranates make an ideal food to add to your diet. The potent antioxidants in pomegranates can relieve inflammation naturally while also preventing free radical damage in cells, and when you add them to healthful apple cider vinegar you create a delicious way to prevent inflammation and treat its symptoms effectively.

Per Serving
Calories: 120 | Fat: 1 g | Protein: 2 g | Sodium: 10 mg
Fiber: 6 g | Carbohydrates: 30 g | Sugar: 22 g

Chapter 11

RECIPES FOR IMPROVED COGNITIVE FUNCTIONING

Regardless of age, we all have days when we feel like our minds are absent—whether we've forgotten our keys, fetched everything at the store except the one thing we initially went for, or forgotten to complete a task that is usually routine. While some of this cognitive dysfunction can be due to simple disruptions in daily life, such as inadequate sleep, skipped meals, emotional stress, hormonal imbalance, or overwhelming workloads, there are a number of instances in which cognitive decline can be an indication of more serious conditions. Whether slight or serious, the underlying issue that contributes to diminished cognitive functioning can be helped with the regular consumption of apple cider vinegar. Combined with nutrient-rich fruits, vegetables, and additions that pack every recipe with brain-boosting vitamins, minerals, and protective antioxidants, the drinks, smoothies, and tonics in this chapter are specifically designed to maximize the benefit to the brain while providing the body's supporting systems with all of the essentials. With these delicious recipes, the days of absentmindedness, forgetfulness, and cognitive decline can be left in the past, and a future filled with focus, productivity, and clarity can be yours.

COCO-CHOCO-CHERRY LATTE

Serves 2

INGREDIENTS

1 tablespoon apple cider vinegar
1 tablespoon coconut oil
2 cups pitted cherries
2 ounces dark chocolate, shredded
2 cups coffee prepared with purified
    water (pH-balanced), chilled

---

1 Combine all the ingredients in
    a large blender.

2 Blend the ingredients on high
    until thoroughly combined and
    frothy.

3 Consume immediately or store
    tightly sealed and unrefriger-
    ated up to 4 hours.

KEY INGREDIENT: Cherries

Cherries contain a number of nutrients that work hard to maintain the health of cells, organs, tissues, and joints and reduce the threat of cognitive decline. In fact, cherries contain significant amounts of antioxidants as well as melatonin, a hormone that has been credited with slowing the aging process and fighting insomnia and depression. Studies have also shown that the anthocyanins in cherries have strong anti-neurodegenerative properties that protect your brain cells from the oxidative stress that can damage them. Helping to fight off illness and diseases of all kinds, cherries and ACV work synergistically to provide the body with essential nutrients like vitamin C and potent unique enzymes, helping you achieve overall health and natural cognitive improvement.

Per Serving
Calories: 330 | Fat: 19 g | Protein: 4 g | Sodium: 10 mg
Fiber: 6 g | Carbohydrates: 39 g | Sugar: 27 g

BLUEBERRY MUFFIN

Serves 2

INGREDIENTS

1 tablespoon apple cider vinegar
1 tablespoon honey
2 cups blueberries
1 cup rolled oats
2 cups low-fat plain Greek yogurt
1 teaspoon ground cinnamon
1 teaspoon ground nutmeg

1 Combine all the ingredients in a large blender.

2 Blend the ingredients on high until thoroughly combined and frothy.

3 Consume immediately or store tightly sealed and refrigerated up to 4 hours.

KEY INGREDIENT: Oats

Oats provide the body with countless benefits, such as heart health, boosted immunity, and essential proteins—and they are good for your brain too! Oats provide your brain with glucose (the brain's basic fuel), and because oats are a low glycemic index food, they provide a slow and steady rise in blood sugar that lasts for a longer time, giving your brain the power it needs for several hours. Delicious and nutritious, oats are also able to provide the body with cleansing fiber and potent phytochemicals that work in the gut to free the digestive tract, blood, and brain of harmful proteins that create inflammation. With these harsh components removed, the body can work as intended without the interference of harmful conditions such as cognitive malfunctioning. By ensuring that the necessary nutrients are available to the brain for proper processing and functioning, oats and apple cider vinegar work with the other ingredients in this recipe to provide the body with all it needs for improved cognitive functioning.

Per Serving
Calories: 440 | Fat: 8 g | Protein: 29 g | Sodium: 80 mg
Fiber: 8 g | Carbohydrates: 67 g | Sugar: 32 g

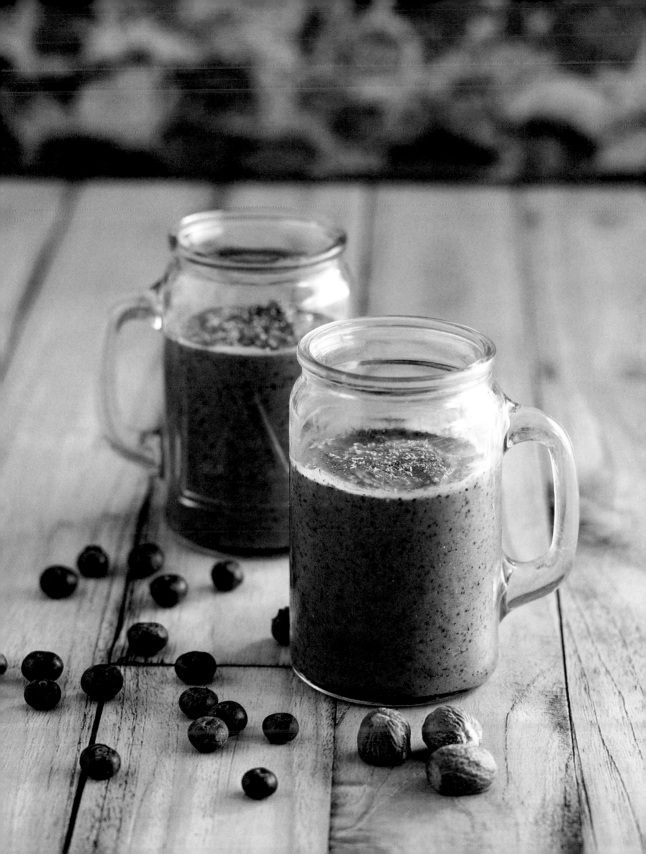

GOJI BERRY BLAST

Serves 2

INGREDIENTS

1 tablespoon apple cider vinegar
1 teaspoon honey
1 cup goji berries
1 medium peach, pitted
1½ cups low-fat vanilla Greek yogurt
½ cup plain kombucha
1 cup ice

---

1 Combine all the ingredients in a large blender.

2 Blend the ingredients on high until thoroughly combined and frothy.

3 Consume immediately or store tightly sealed and refrigerated up to 4 hours.

KEY INGREDIENT: Goji Berries

While not many people are familiar with the sweet, slightly tart fruit that is the goji berry, its restorative capabilities for cognitive cells are significant enough to warrant inclusion in any proactive diet concerning cognitive health. Goji berries are packed with nutrients like ascorbic acid, beta-carotene, lutein, and B and E vitamins, as well as minerals such as calcium, copper, selenium, and zinc. In addition to improving vision and protecting the immune system, the nutrients in goji berries may also insulate the brain from toxic beta-amyloid proteins that can cause Alzheimer's disease. By combining these delightful fruits with antioxidant-abundant peaches; creamy, protein-packed yogurt; and enzyme-rich apple cider vinegar, the goal of this drink is to provide the body and brain with potent antioxidants and phytochemicals that naturally combat cognitive decline. The combination of delicious and nutritious phytochemical-fueled foods like those contained in this refreshing drink makes for a simple snack that fights cognitive decline naturally.

Per Serving
Calories: 330 | Fat: 3.5 g | Protein: 24 g | Sodium: 200 mg
Fiber: 7 g | Carbohydrates: 53 g | Sugar: 36 g

SAVORY SPICED TOMATO

Serves 2

INGREDIENTS

1 tablespoon apple cider vinegar
1 clove garlic, peeled
¼ cup peeled and chopped red
  onion
2 large tomatoes, chopped
1 cup spinach leaves
2 cups purified water (pH-balanced)

1 Combine all the ingredients in
   a large blender.

2 Blend the ingredients on high
   until thoroughly combined and
   frothy.

3 Consume immediately or store
   tightly sealed and unrefrigerated up to 4 hours.

KEY INGREDIENT: Red Onions

Red onions contain potent antioxidant-rich enzymes that can fill any snack, smoothie, salad, or entrée with preventative properties that help combat cognitive decline. Among other nutrients, onions contain vitamin C, vitamin B_6, and manganese, all of which have been shown to improve the health of your nervous system and brain. In fact, studies have shown that eating onions can help when the brain has been damaged by a stroke or a blood clot. Red onions also provide the body with unique compounds, such as allicin, that move through the body with powerful cleansing capabilities that focus specifically on inflammatory proteins. Helping to combat the buildup of unhealthy inflammatory compounds that can wreak havoc on the brain cells and nervous system, red onions clear the path for healthy antioxidants to do their work. While eating red onions in salads can be slightly overwhelming to the senses, combining them with apple cider vinegar and tomatoes makes for a slightly spicy drink that opens the sinuses but is not overpowering. With this drink you can contribute to the fight against the onset of inflammation-related illness that can adversely affect your mental processes and cognitive functioning.

Per Serving
Calories: 44 | Fat: 0.5 g | Protein: 2 g | Sodium: 25 mg
Fiber: 3 g | Carbohydrates: 10 g | Sugar: 6 g

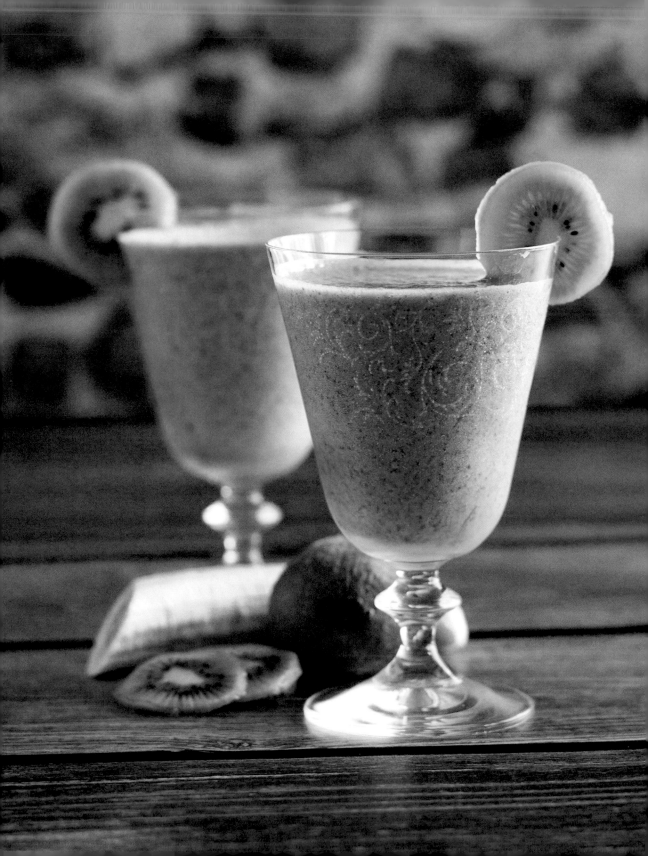

GREAT GREEN KIWI

Serves 2

INGREDIENTS

1 tablespoon apple cider vinegar

2 medium kiwis, peeled

1 medium banana, peeled and frozen

1 cup spinach leaves

1 cup ice

2 cups purified water (pH-balanced)

---

1 Combine all the ingredients in a large blender.

2 Blend the ingredients on high until thoroughly combined and frothy.

3 Consume immediately or store tightly sealed and unrefrigerated up to 4 hours.

KEY INGREDIENT: Kiwi

Rich in potent vitamin C, kiwi not only acts to support the body's natural immune defenses, but it also works to fight cognitive complications too. In addition to high amounts of vitamin C, kiwis contain close to twenty vital nutrients, including vitamins A, K, and B, potassium, copper, folate, and fiber. They are also packed with antioxidants that help prevent the effects of oxidation on the brain. While the vitamins, minerals, and antioxidants of the kiwi work at supporting a healthy brain and nervous system, the enzymes of apple cider vinegar remove harmful proteins from the bloodstream. These nutrient-dense foods work to promote overall health and well-being, and the protective abilities of their antioxidants make this ACV drink an effective choice for anyone who wants to fight cognitive decline naturally.

Per Serving
Calories: 100 | Fat: 0.5 g | Protein: 2 g | Sodium: 15 mg
Fiber: 4 g | Carbohydrates: 25 g | Sugar: 14 g

SWEET SQUASH

Serves 2

INGREDIENTS

1 tablespoon apple cider vinegar
2 cups roasted, peeled, and
    chopped acorn squash
1 cup nonfat vanilla Greek yogurt
1 cup unsweetened vanilla almond
    milk
1 teaspoon ground cinnamon
1 teaspoon ground nutmeg
½ teaspoon ground cloves
1 cup ice

1 Combine all the ingredients in
a large blender.

2 Blend the ingredients on high
until thoroughly combined and
frothy.

3 Consume immediately or store
tightly sealed and refrigerated
up to 4 hours.

KEY INGREDIENT: Acorn Squash

Acorn squash is a lycopene-rich food with a sweet, earthy taste that adds an incomparable flavor to almost any smoothie, drink, salad, or entrée in which it stars. With plentiful phytochemicals and antioxidants that play a major role in the prevention of cognitive decline, acorn squash and apple cider vinegar combine to provide the body with supportive properties that not only cleanse the blood and promote proper nutrient absorption and distribution but also work to remove caustic inflammatory proteins from the brain and bloodstream. This quick and easy ACV drink emphasizes the preventative properties and health-promoting phytochemicals of a natural vegetable like acorn squash and should be included in your daily diet.

Per Serving
Calories: 230 | Fat: 2.5 g | Protein: 13 g | Sodium: 140 mg
Fiber: 11 g | Carbohydrates: 45 g | Sugar: 19 g

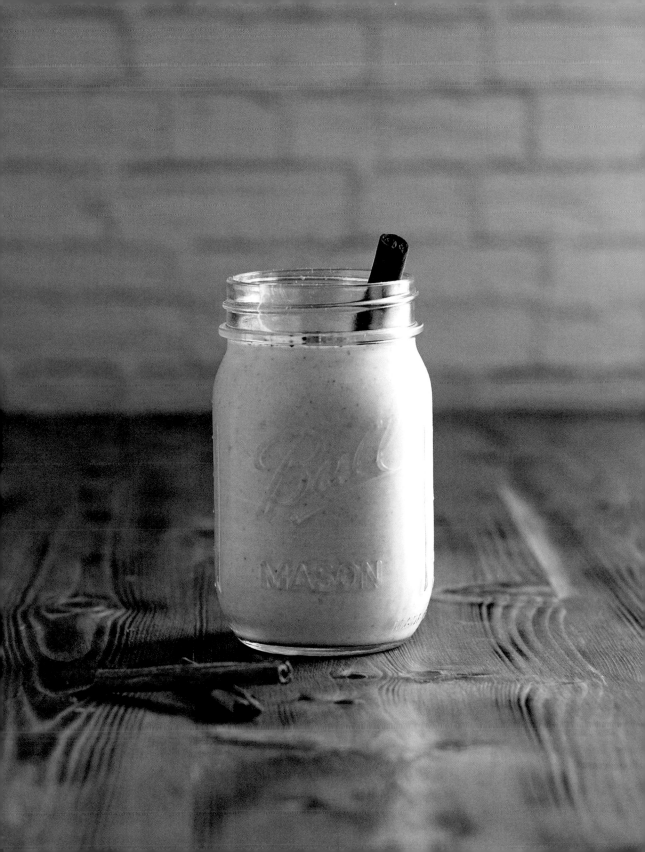

SPICED ZUCCHINI CARROT

Serves 2

INGREDIENTS

- 1 tablespoon apple cider vinegar
- 1 tablespoon peeled and grated fresh gingerroot
- 1 tablespoon honey
- 1 medium zucchini, chopped
- 1 large carrot, greens removed
- 1 cup spinach leaves
- 2 cups purified water (pH-balanced)

1 Combine all the ingredients in a large blender.

2 Blend the ingredients on high until thoroughly combined and frothy.

3 Consume immediately or store tightly sealed and unrefrigerated up to 4 hours.

KEY INGREDIENT: Zucchini

While many consider zucchini to be "tasteless," this moisturizing green vegetable has notable health benefits, including helping with weight loss, improving eye health, guarding against asthma, and helping to lower cholesterol. Zucchini contains vitamins A, C, B_6, and K, folate, and manganese. In terms of cognitive health, the vitamin C in zucchini is essential to the production of neurotransmitters, which affect your ability to focus, concentrate, and remember. Vitamin C also fights the free radical damage that the brain is susceptible to. When considering clean, whole foods that should be included in a diet focused on protecting and maximizing cognitive functioning, remember zucchini and apple cider vinegar for their shared abilities in helping prevent cognitive decline, disease, or malfunction simply and naturally.

Per Serving
Calories: 70 | Fat: 0.5 g | Protein: 2 g | Sodium: 45 mg
Fiber: 2 g | Carbohydrates: 16 g | Sugar: 13 g

Chapter 12

RECIPES FOR STRESS REDUCTION

Stress is a natural part of life that arises in every person's day at some point. Whatever the cause of the stress, the body reacts with hormones and biochemicals that stimulate the body and brain. Whether the stress is a result of something minimal, such as being late, or intense, such as fearing for one's safety, the toll that chronic stress can have on the body and mind is far more detrimental than you might think. Wreaking havoc on the heart rate, blood pressure, digestive processes, mental functions, nervous system communication, and hormone production, chronic stress can lead to anxiety, depression, weakened immunity, and a variety of chronic illnesses and conditions that can easily be avoided. By implementing a daily apple cider vinegar regimen that provides the body with supportive enzymes, nutrients, and antioxidants, the body and brain can begin and sustain a healing process that helps better regulate stress. With natural fruits and vegetables that add plentiful benefits to your delicious and nutritious stress-reducing ACV drinks, you'll be sipping your way to less stress in no time!

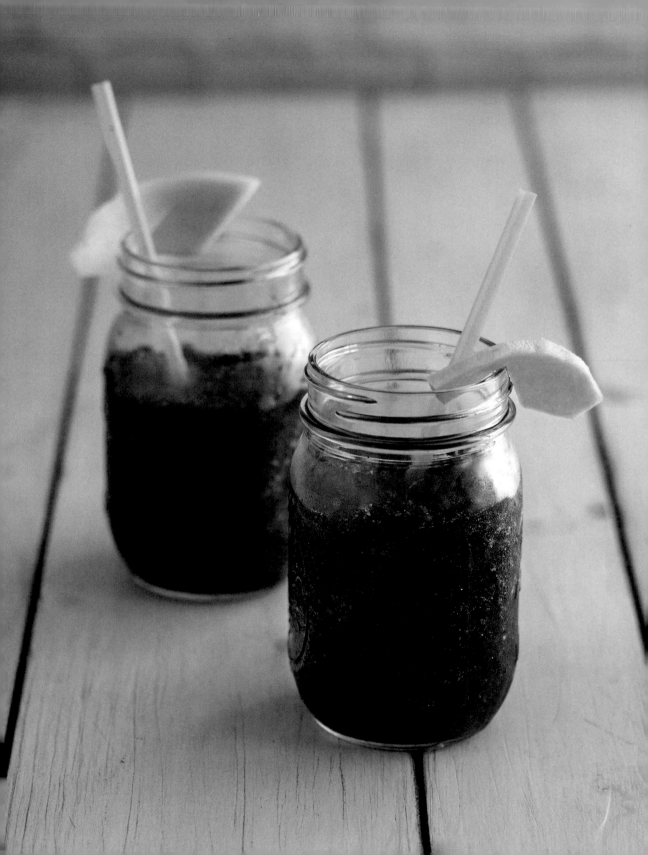

BLUE CANTALOUPE CHAMOMILE WITH ACV

Serves 2

INGREDIENTS

1 tablespoon apple cider vinegar

1 tablespoon honey

1 cup blueberries

1 cup chopped cantaloupe

1 cup ice

2 cups chamomile tea prepared
with purified water (pH-balanced),
cooled

---

1 Combine all the ingredients in
   a large blender.

2 Blend the ingredients on high
   until thoroughly combined and
   frothy.

3 Consume immediately or store
   tightly sealed and unrefrigerated up to 4 hours.

KEY INGREDIENT: Chamomile Tea

Chamomile tea has been widely recommended to anyone hoping to reduce stress. Caffeine-free and packed with phytochemicals that soothe the body's fight-or-flight response, chamomile tea has a calming effect on both body and mind. Chamomile tea can increase the serotonin and melatonin levels in your body, which can help eliminate worry and stress while making you feel calmer and less anxious. Chamomile tea also helps fight insomnia, a symptom of stress, by helping you fall asleep faster and waking up more refreshed. With its phytochemicals that contribute to the body's natural stress-relieving hormone production, chamomile tea can be combined with nutrient-dense clean foods for a healing diet that not only relieves stress but also protects the body from degrading toxins. Light and crisp, chamomile tea makes for the perfect pairing with apple cider vinegar.

Per Serving

Calories: 100 | Fat: 0.5 g | Protein: 1 g | Sodium: 15 mg
Fiber: 3 g | Carbohydrates: 26 g | Sugar: 22 g

SWEET BERRY KOMBUCHA TEA WITH ACV

Serves 2
INGREDIENTS

1 tablespoon apple cider vinegar
1 tablespoon honey
2 cups hulled strawberries
1 tablespoon fresh mint leaves
2 cups plain kombucha

1 Combine all the ingredients in a large blender.
2 Blend the ingredients on high until thoroughly combined and frothy.
3 Consume immediately or store tightly sealed and unrefrigerated up to 4 hours.

KEY INGREDIENT: Mint

Stress hormones like adrenaline and cortisol serve an important purpose in times of true danger, but they can also cause difficult disturbances in everyday life through a variety of symptoms. From stomachaches to insomnia, the results of the body's natural fight-or-flight response can be unpleasant to say the least. Herbs like mint have a calming effect on the mind and body. The menthol in mint helps to relax the muscles, while the herb's nutrients and antioxidants offer nutrition and protection against cell damage. When combined with fruits, vegetables, and enzyme-rich elixirs like apple cider vinegar, mint can add an element of refreshment that not only improves overall health but also reduces stress levels naturally.

Per Serving
Calories: 110 | Fat: 0.5 g | Protein: 1 g | Sodium: 15 mg
Fiber: 3 g | Carbohydrates: 27 g | Sugar: 18 g

MINTY MELON

Serves 2
INGREDIENTS

1 tablespoon apple cider vinegar
1 tablespoon maple syrup
1 cup fresh mint leaves
2 cups chopped honeydew melon
1 cup purified water (pH-balanced)

1 Combine all the ingredients in a large blender.
2 Blend the ingredients on high until thoroughly combined and frothy.
3 Consume immediately or store tightly sealed and unrefrigerated up to 4 hours.

KEY INGREDIENT: Honeydew Melon

Rich in vitamin C and potassium, green honeydew melon makes for a delicious and nutritious moisturizing ingredient that not only soothes skin and improves immunity but also adds stress-relieving phytochemicals to any dish you create. The vitamin C helps to flush out stress hormones like cortisol, while the potassium helps to regulate blood pressure levels. So, if you are feeling stressed or overwhelmed, whip up this sweet and invigorating drink. The simple blending of apple cider vinegar and honeydew can promote healthy hormone maintenance and overall well-being for all-natural stress relief that tastes great!

Per Serving
Calories: 100 | Fat: 0.5 g | Protein: 1 g | Sodium: 40 mg
Fiber: 2 g | Carbohydrates: 24 g | Sugar: 20 g

SPICY PEACH CHILLER

Serves 2

INGREDIENTS

1 tablespoon apple cider vinegar

1 tablespoon honey

2 medium peaches, pitted

1 teaspoon nutmeg

1 teaspoon peeled and grated fresh gingerroot

2 cups green tea prepared with purified water (pH-balanced), cooled

---

1 Combine all the ingredients in a large blender.

2 Blend the ingredients on high until thoroughly combined and frothy.

3 Consume immediately or store tightly sealed and unrefrigerated up to 4 hours.

KEY INGREDIENT: Ginger

Ginger has been used as a healing ingredient around the world for thousands of years. With unique phytochemicals called gingerols that travel throughout the brain and body to rectify imbalances, ginger works wonders when it comes to stress reduction. Helping to maintain a healthy balance of the stress hormones adrenaline and cortisol, as well as the "feel-good" neurotransmitters dopamine and serotonin, ginger is able to purge the brain and bloodstream of harmful toxins that can adversely affect the body's natural hormone production and distribution. Ginger is also excellent for soothing certain symptoms of stress, such as indigestion, making this ACV drink a must for natural stress relief.

Per Serving

Calories: 100 | Fat: 1 g | Protein: 2 g | Sodium: 3 mg
Fiber: 3 g | Carbohydrates: 24 g | Sugar: 21 g

RASPBERRY-GINGER WITH LIME FIZZ

Serves 2
INGREDIENTS

1 tablespoon apple cider vinegar
1 tablespoon peeled and chopped
   fresh gingerroot
2 cups raspberries
1 medium lime, peeled and
   deseeded
1 cup ice
1 cup white tea prepared with purified water (pH-balanced), cooled
1 cup seltzer water

1 In a large blender, combine all
   the ingredients except seltzer
   water.

2 Blend the ingredients on high
   until thoroughly combined and
   frothy.

3 Stir in seltzer water and continue blending until all ingredients are thoroughly combined.

4 Consume immediately or store
   tightly sealed and unrefrigerated up to 4 hours.

KEY INGREDIENT: White Tea

Like chamomile tea, white tea contributes unique phyto-chemicals and antioxidants to delicious and nutritious recipes like this one. White tea is a delicate variety because it is so minimally processed. It is harvested before the tea plant's leaves fully open, and then the leaves are quickly dried so they do not oxidize as long as other kinds of tea leaves. White tea is also more calming than other kinds of tea because it contains less caffeine (which stimulates the brain, giving you a jittery feeling). By adding white tea to a recipe, anyone hoping to achieve stress relief can do so easily and health-fully. While some of the ingredients may seem to contradict one another in taste or texture, this particular combination of clean foods, tea, and apple cider vinegar fulfills nutrient needs while replenishing and rehydrating the cells and help-ing to improve hormonal balance. This recipe can ensure that the entire body benefits from countless nutrients, helping to achieve an overall sense of calm and well-being. Quick and easy, simple and delicious, this ACV drink is one that will help reduce stress effectively and naturally.

Per Serving
Calories: 80 | Fat: 1 g | Protein: 2 g | Sodium: 4 mg
Fiber: 9 g | Carbohydrates: 18 g | Sugar: 6 g

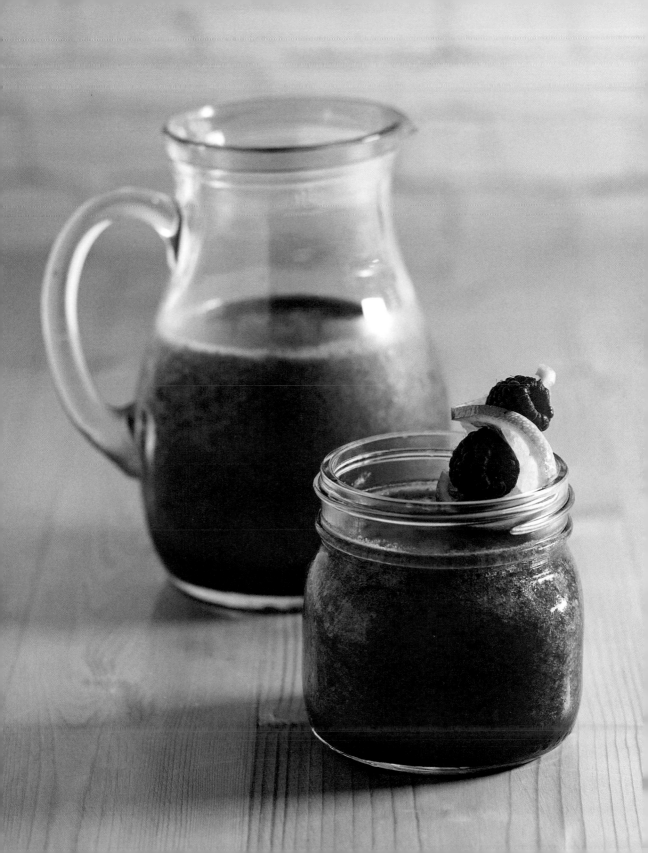

KALE APPLE WITH ACV

Serves 2

INGREDIENTS

1 tablespoon apple cider vinegar

3 large kale leaves with ribs removed, chopped

2 medium Granny Smith apples, cored

1 teaspoon ground cinnamon

¼ teaspoon ground cloves

2 cups organic apple juice (not from concentrate)

---

1 Combine all the ingredients, except the apple juice, in a large blender.

2 Blend the ingredients on high until thoroughly combined and frothy.

3 Add the apple juice gradually until desired consistency is reached.

4 Consume immediately or store tightly sealed and unrefrigerated up to 4 hours.

KEY INGREDIENT: Apples

Apples are a sweet, slightly tart ingredient that can add a unique flavor sensation to any dish. When combined with soothing spices that calm the senses and provide the body with potent phytochemicals, apples become key in the battle for stress relief. Apples contain a unique flavonoid, quercetin, which works synergistically with the apple's fiber to cleanse the gut of impurities and undigested bits of food that can disrupt digestive processes and interfere with hormone production and distribution. By consuming apples regularly, you can easily achieve more balanced hormone levels. Adding whole foods like apples to apple cider vinegar drink recipes such as this one can create a sensational combination that works throughout the body to improve immunity, maximize metabolic functioning, boost cognition, regulate hormones, and reduce stress naturally. In a matter of days, a clarifying diet of clean foods and drinks made with naturally stress-reducing foods can transform your health and minimize your stress levels.

Per Serving

Calories: 260 | Fat: 1 g | Protein: 5 g | Sodium: 60 mg
Fiber: 9 g | Carbohydrates: 61 g | Sugar: 48 g

GRAPEFRUIT-KIWI TEA WITH A TWIST

Serves 2
INGREDIENTS

1 tablespoon apple cider vinegar

2 medium pink grapefruits, peeled and deseeded

2 medium kiwis, peeled

1 tablespoon peeled and grated fresh gingerroot

1½ cups chamomile tea prepared with purified water (pH-balanced), cooled

½ cup plain kombucha

---

1 Combine all the ingredients in a large blender.

2 Blend the ingredients on high until thoroughly combined and frothy.

3 Consume immediately or store tightly sealed and unrefrigerated up to 4 hours.

KEY INGREDIENT: Kiwi

Kiwis are a sweet treat that can make any delicious drink even tastier. In addition to kiwis' amazing flavor, these beautiful green fruits add an enormous amount of vitamin C as well as unique phytochemicals and antioxidants that work to purge toxins and inhibitory compounds from the body. When the body is free of these agents, its natural stress-relieving mechanisms are able to work as intended and protect against the negative effects of stress. In addition, kiwis have been proved to fight insomnia, a common symptom of stress, and have been linked to substantial improvements in both sleep quality and quantity. When kiwis are combined with ingredients such as citrus, ginger, kombucha, and chamomile tea, their health benefits become even more powerful and ensure that the body's nutritional needs for everything from energy production to immunity are met. When all is well for nutritional provisions throughout body, there is a far less incidence of stress and stress-related symptoms, such as lethargy and anxiety. So utilize the powers of apple cider vinegar and kiwi in this delicious drink to reduce your stress levels naturally.

Per Serving
Calories: 160 | Fat: 1 g | Protein: 3 g | Sodium: 5 mg
Fiber: 6 g | Carbohydrates: 40 g | Sugar: 24 g

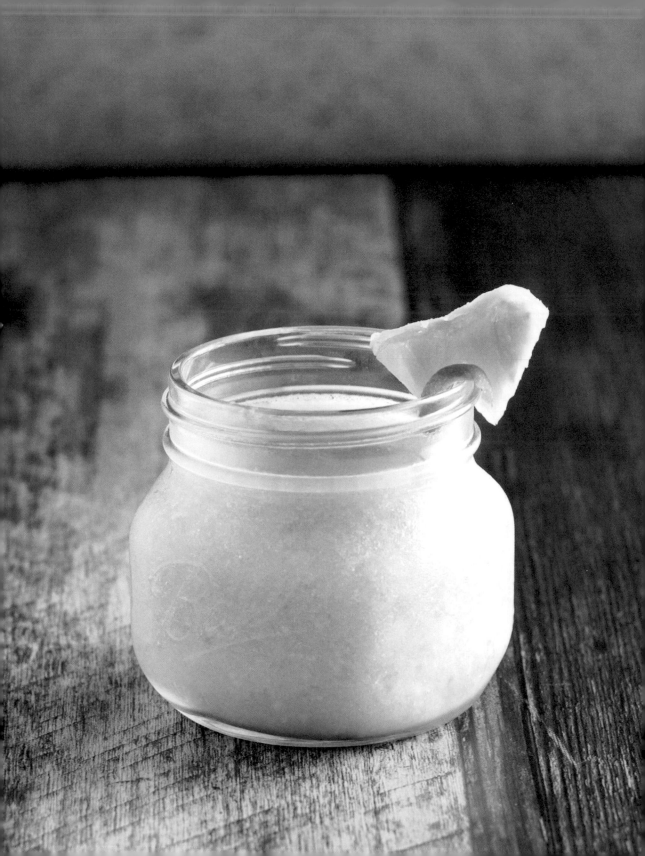

MANGO TANGO

Serves 2

INGREDIENTS

1 tablespoon apple cider vinegar

1 large mango, peeled and pitted

1 medium orange, peeled and deseeded

½ cup chopped pineapple

1 cup ice

1 cup dandelion tea prepared with purified water (pH-balanced), cooled

½ cup plain kombucha

---

1 Combine all the ingredients in a large blender.

2 Blend the ingredients on high until thoroughly combined and frothy.

3 Consume immediately or store tightly sealed and unrefrigerated up to 4 hours.

KEY INGREDIENT: Mango

Mango is a nutritious and delicious fruit that is rich in flavor and nutrients. A plentiful source of vitamin A, B vitamins, and phytochemicals like folate, mangos can be added to almost any recipe for an impressive improvement in taste and a boost in stress-reducing nutrients. The free radical–fighting antioxidants in mangos travel through the body and fend off harmful agents and toxins that can cause damage to cells. Mangos also contain magnesium, which helps muscles like the heart relax more fully so it can recover better between beats. It also helps lower blood pressure and help you feel more relaxed. While tasting sweet and delicious, this astounding fruit works to boost brain function as well, naturally supporting the brain and its provision of stress-reducing hormones. With the addition of apple cider vinegar and other clean, whole foods, this drink can help you reduce your stress naturally with adequate stores of brain-boosting nutrition.

Per Serving

Calories: 140 | Fat: 0.5 g | Protein: 2 g | Sodium: 5 mg
Fiber: 4 g | Carbohydrates: 34 g | Sugar: 28 g

Chapter 13

RECIPES FOR MEN'S HEALTH

Regardless of their age, men have to consider maintaining a level of health that will help them live longer and more happily—in ways that differ greatly from the approaches taken by the opposite sex. For men, the heart, prostate, lungs, and muscles can fall victim to specific kinds of deterioration over time, resulting in serious health issues that can complicate or threaten life. With a balanced, healthy diet packed with nutrient-dense fruits, vegetables, grains, and other additions, like apple cider vinegar, the body's cells, organs, and systems can be supported and optimized. Helping to prevent the carcinogenic effects of free radicals, apple cider vinegar's nutrients and enzymes work to scavenge harmful toxins and protect the body from dangerous changes that can cause serious illness. Each of the delicious and nutritious ACV-based drinks in this chapter can help a man of any age protect himself from the detrimental effects of nutritional neglect and lifestyle choices.

SPICED GREENS AND FIGS

Serves 2

INGREDIENTS

1 tablespoon apple cider vinegar
2 medium figs
1 teaspoon peeled and grated fresh gingerroot
2 cups spinach leaves
2 cups purified water (pH-balanced)

1 In a large blender, combine the vinegar, figs, ginger, and spinach.

2 Blend the ingredients until thoroughly combined and frothy.

3 Add the water gradually and continue blending until desired consistency is reached.

4 Consume immediately or store tightly sealed and unrefrigerated up to 4 hours.

KEY INGREDIENT: Figs

While flavor combinations such as figs and ginger may seem a little strange, this ingredient list is the perfect one for any man seeking an energy boost in a glass. The phytochemicals and antioxidants in figs have been used to fight sexual dysfunctions in men such as sterility, endurance issues, and erectile dysfunction. And while they are not actually an aphrodisiac, the large amounts of vitamins and minerals contained in figs will give you a sudden boost of energy and stamina that could feel like a sexual surge. Figs also work to prevent constipation, lower cholesterol levels, control diabetes, and strengthen bones. Helping to regulate hormones, amplify the effects of antioxidants against free radical changes in cells, and maintain muscle mass over a lifetime, the essential nutrients provided in this apple cider vinegar drink recipe can be life-changing, especially for men.

Per Serving
Calories: 50 | Fat: 0.5 g | Protein: 1 g | Sodium: 25 mg
Fiber: 2 g | Carbohydrates: 11 g | Sugar: 8 g

PEACHY POMEGRANATE FIZZ

Serves 2

INGREDIENTS

1 tablespoon apple cider vinegar
1 cup pomegranate arils (jewels)
½ cup plain kombucha
½ medium peach, pitted
1 cup ice
2 cups seltzer water

1   In a large blender, combine the vinegar, pomegranate jewels, kombucha, peach, and ice.

2   Blend the ingredients until thoroughly combined and frothy.

3   Add seltzer water gradually and continue blending until desired consistency is reached.

4   Consume immediately or store tightly sealed and unrefrigerated up to 4 hours. Shake well to revive fizz before serving.

KEY INGREDIENT: Pomegranate

While the pomegranate's sweet, deep-red jewels can add sensational flavor to any drink or dish, this delightful fruit provides countless health benefits, especially for men. Studies have shown that pomegranates are able to help protect the prostate against free radical damage while cleansing the colon naturally and effectively. Pomegranates also help with erectile dysfunctions, fight prostate and lung cancer, and reduce the risk of type 2 diabetes. In this drink, the health-boosting effects of the pomegranate join forces with the enzymes naturally occurring in apple cider vinegar that work to expel toxins, cleanse the blood, support neuron activity, and increase energy production. At any age, men who seek all-natural methods to achieve greater overall health will benefit immensely with every sip of this ACV-and-pomegranate drink.

Per Serving
Calories: 90 | Fat: 1 g | Protein: 2 g | Sodium: 5 mg
Fiber: 4 g | Carbohydrates: 22 g | Sugar: 16 g

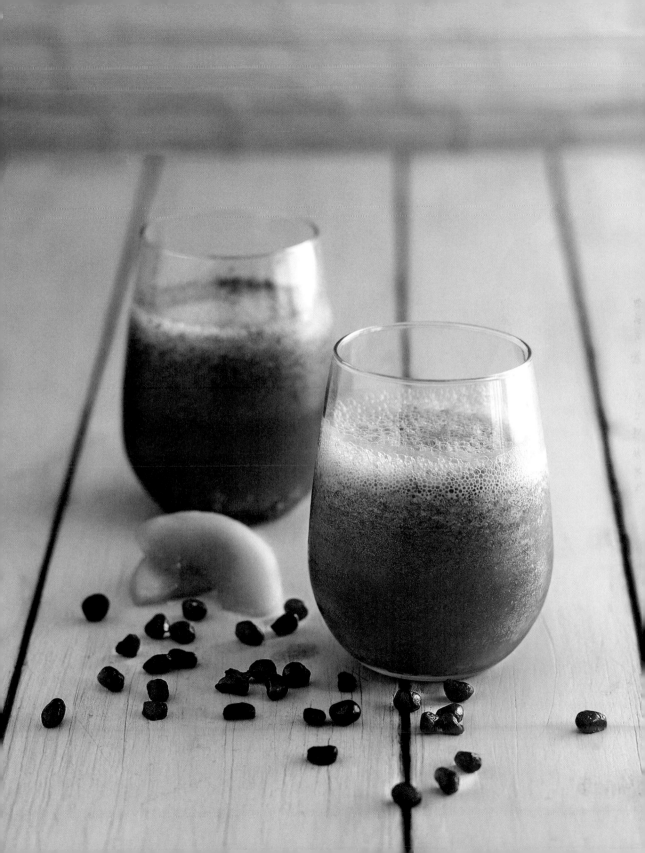

SPICY SALSA AND CREAM

Serves 2

INGREDIENTS

1 tablespoon apple cider vinegar
3 medium tomatoes, chopped
½ small red onion, peeled and
    chopped
1 small jalapeño, deseeded and
    chopped
½ cup nonfat Greek yogurt
2 cups purified water (pH-balanced)

1   Combine all the ingredients in
    a large blender.

2   Blend the ingredients on high
    until thoroughly combined and
    frothy.

3   Consume immediately or store
    tightly sealed and refrigerated
    up to 4 hours.

KEY INGREDIENT: Jalapeño

Fighting off illness, promoting heart health, and improving energy stores through maximized metabolic processes, the jalapeño's phytochemical, capsaicin, is able to work wonders in males of any age. With delicious flavors that create a spicy, savory sensation, the ingredients in this apple cider vinegar drink provide powerful vitamins such as A and C; minerals such as potassium, iron, and magnesium; phytochemicals; and antioxidants so that the body and brain can thrive as naturally intended. Regardless of current condition, any man hoping to achieve better health and improve his quality of life can use this recipe to gain protective, preventative, and health-promoting nutrients that satisfy and exceed nutritional needs.

Per Serving
Calories: 80 | Fat: 0.5 g | Protein: 8 g | Sodium: 45 mg
Fiber: 3 g | Carbohydrates: 12 g | Sugar: 7 g

CREAMY BLUEBERRY CRUMBLE

Serves 2

INGREDIENTS

1 tablespoon apple cider vinegar
½ cup low-fat granola
2 cups blueberries
2 cups nonfat plain Greek yogurt
1 teaspoon ground cinnamon
¼ teaspoon ground cloves
1 cup ice
½ cup purified water (pH-balanced)

---

1 In a large blender, combine the vinegar, granola, blueberries, yogurt, cinnamon, cloves, and ice.

2 Blend the ingredients on high until thoroughly combined and frothy.

3 Add the water gradually and continue blending until desired consistency is reached.

4 Consume immediately or store tightly sealed and refrigerated up to 4 hours.

KEY INGREDIENT: Greek Yogurt

While a blueberry muffin may sound like a great idea, most of the blueberry-packed foods available in markets and restaurants can be laden with sugars, unhealthy fats, and unnatural preservatives. By whipping up this quick and easy yogurt-and-ACV drink that contains all of the nutrients a man needs, anyone hoping to achieve greater overall health and extend and improve his life can find success naturally. The Greek yogurt supplies ample amounts of protein for energy production, hormone balance, and muscle mass protection, as well as calcium to strengthen bones. Since most men, especially older men, do not get the recommended 1,000 mg of calcium a day, this yogurt drink is a quick and easy way to boost your calcium intake so your bones and body stay strong and protected.

Per Serving
Calories: 370 | Fat: 9 g | Protein: 28 g | Sodium: 95 mg
Fiber: 7 g | Carbohydrates: 47 g | Sugar: 28 g

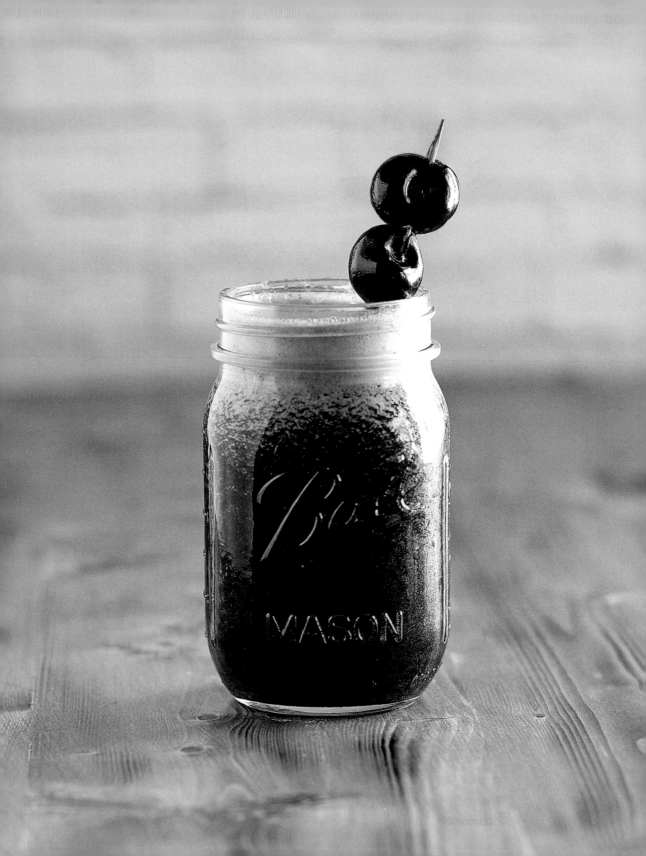

HOT AND SPICY SWEETNESS

Serves 2
INGREDIENTS

1 tablespoon apple cider vinegar
1 teaspoon peeled and grated fresh
  gingerroot
¼ teaspoon cayenne pepper
2 cups pitted cherries
1 cup ice
½ cup plain kombucha
1½ cups purified water (pH-balanced)

---

1 In a large blender, combine
   the vinegar, ginger, cayenne,
   cherries, ice, and kombucha.

2 Blend the ingredients on high
   until thoroughly combined and
   frothy.

3 Add the water gradually and
   continue blending until desired
   consistency is reached.

4 Consume immediately or store
   tightly sealed and unrefrigerated up to 4 hours.

KEY INGREDIENT: Cherries

Cherries contain massive amounts of naturally occurring phytochemicals and antioxidants that are able to work with other clean ingredients, such as ginger, in preventing illness and promoting health. By consuming vitamin C–rich cherries in combination with additional all-natural ingredients, men seeking sustained energy, improved focus and cognition, and better cholesterol levels can achieve their goals healthfully and naturally. The phytosterols in cherries help to regulate cholesterol, potentially lowering the risk for the number one killer of men: heart disease. The antioxidants quercetin and anthocyanin also fight against heart disease while lowering men's risk for cancer. A cherry-packed diet that includes enzyme-rich elixirs such as apple cider vinegar can satisfy the body's nutritional needs and eliminate various dysfunctions in the male brain and body naturally.

Per Serving
Calories: 110 | Fat: 0.5 g | Protein: 2 g | Sodium: 5 mg
Fiber: 3 g | Carbohydrates: 27 g | Sugar: 20 g

AMPED APPLE-STRAWBERRY-BANANA WITH GREENS

Serves 2

INGREDIENTS

1 tablespoon apple cider vinegar
½ medium Fuji apple, cored
½ cup hulled strawberries
1 medium banana, peeled and
    frozen
1 cup spinach leaves
2 cups purified water (pH-balanced)

1   In a large blender, combine
    the vinegar, apple, strawber-
    ries, banana, and spinach.

2   Blend the ingredients on high
    until thoroughly combined and
    frothy.

3   Add the water gradually and
    continue blending until desired
    consistency is reached.

4   Consume immediately or store
    tightly sealed and unrefriger-
    ated up to 4 hours.

KEY INGREDIENT: Banana

Bananas are one of the most amazing fruits for men's health. Supporting the brain with B vitamins, vitamin C, and potassium, bananas also protect the rest of the body with antioxidants that help prevent free radical damage in every cell, tissue, and organ. Simultaneously supporting the communication between neurons, stimulating brain activity and energy production, and increasing immunity, the nutrients in bananas combine with apple cider vinegar's enzymes to cleanse the blood, balance hormone levels, and maintain muscle mass over time. ACV drinks with banana can transform a man's health in a matter of weeks. For a male of any age who is in search of the perfect pick-me-up, this banana ACV drink is a winner!

Per Serving
Calories: 100 | Fat: 0.5 g | Protein: 1 g | Sodium: 15 mg
Fiber: 4 g | Carbohydrates: 24 g | Sugar: 15 g

SWEET BANANA, CHOCOLATE, AND CHERRY

Serves 2

INGREDIENTS

1 tablespoon apple cider vinegar

1 cup pitted cherries

1 medium banana, peeled and frozen

1 ounce dark chocolate

½ cup plain kombucha

1½ cups purified water (pH-balanced)

1 In a large blender, combine the vinegar, cherries, banana, chocolate, and kombucha.

2 Blend the ingredients on high until thoroughly combined and frothy.

3 Add the water gradually and continue blending until desired consistency is reached.

4 Consume immediately or store tightly sealed and unrefrigerated up to 4 hours.

KEY INGREDIENT: Kombucha

With enzymes and acids that naturally arise during the fermentation process, kombucha is able to work throughout the body to provide the cells, organs, and systems with all types of support. This unique beverage not only protects against degradation and damage but also helps to maintain healthy levels of sugars in the bloodstream, hormones in the brain, and flora in the gut. With all of these benefits, it's no wonder that adding nutritious, whole foods and enzyme-rich apple cider vinegar to kombucha can make for a winning men's health drink. Maximizing energy production, cognitive processes, and sexual stamina, kombucha can improve any man's quality of life simply and easily—especially when combined with the healthy and flavorful ingredients in this recipe.

Per Serving

Calories: 190 | Fat: 6 g | Protein: 3 g | Sodium: 10 mg
Fiber: 5 g | Carbohydrates: 34 g | Sugar: 21 g

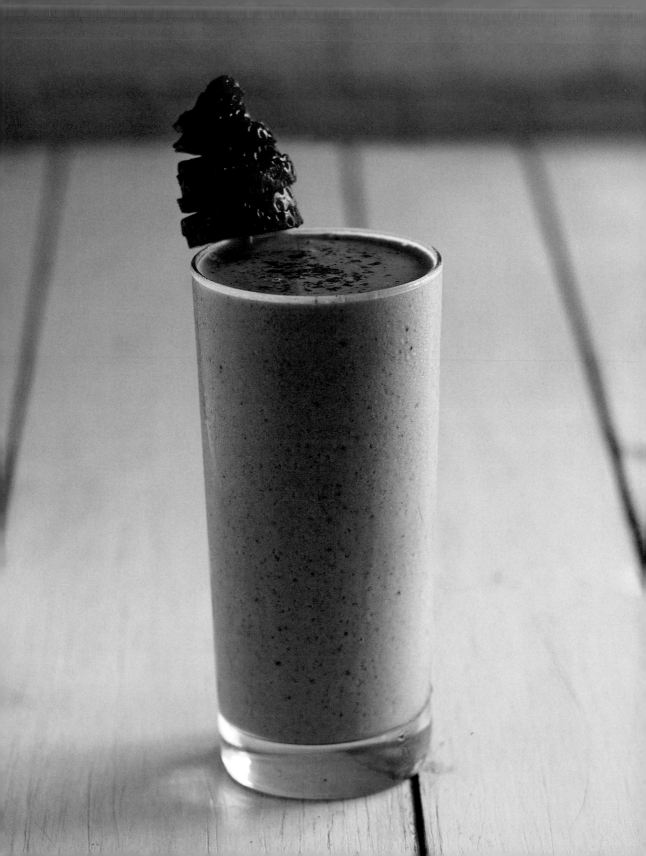

TEMPTING TWO FRUIT CREAM

Serves 2

INGREDIENTS

1 tablespoon apple cider vinegar
¼ teaspoon ground cloves
1 cup hulled strawberries
1 medium peach, pitted
1 cup low-fat plain Greek yogurt
1 cup ice
1 cup purified water (pH-balanced)

1 In a large blender, combine the vinegar, cloves, strawberries, peach, yogurt, and ice.

2 Blend the ingredients on high until thoroughly combined and frothy.

3 Add the water gradually and continue blending until desired consistency is reached.

4 Consume immediately or store tightly sealed and refrigerated up to 4 hours.

KEY INGREDIENT: Peaches

Rich in antioxidants, peaches provide the body's cells with protective properties that can't be beat. Traveling throughout the bloodstream, peaches' antioxidants scour the body and brain for free radicals that compromise the health and functioning of cells. With the incidence of cancers and other serious diseases on the rise every year, men should be consuming adequate amounts of nutrients and antioxidants that naturally combat these caustic changes. In addition, peaches and other stone fruits have been shown to help fight metabolic syndrome. Metabolic syndrome is a medical condition in which obesity and inflammation lead to serious health issues, and is more likely to develop in men than women. By enjoying vibrant peaches and berries, as in this recipe, the average man is able to satisfy his needs for nutrition while also safeguarding his cells, organs, and systems against harm. Protective prevention can be found in every last sip of this delicious drink!

Per Serving
Calories: 140 | Fat: 3 g | Protein: 12 g | Sodium: 40 mg
Fiber: 3 g | Carbohydrates: 17 g | Sugar: 14 g

Chapter 14

RECIPES FOR WOMEN'S HEALTH

Women's health is an issue that seems to be making news daily. With the increasing awareness of breast cancer, the prevalence of sexually transmitted diseases such as HPV, and hormonal fluctuations that can adversely affect everyday life, it's important for women to educate themselves on the preventative measures that can be taken to promote their health proactively, effectively, and naturally. Extensive studies have revealed the protective properties contained within natural foods, prompting many women to make smarter dietary choices that benefit their overall health, such as consuming apple cider vinegar. With the unique recipes in this chapter, women can enjoy sweet and savory combinations of delicious produce and ACV that combat free radicals, promote natural metabolic functions, support digestive health, and activate anti-aging capabilities naturally. Utilizing the essential nutrients that the female body needs to thrive, these satisfying culinary concoctions can help every woman enjoy life to the fullest!

MELON-KIWI-BERRY SPRITZER

Serves 2

INGREDIENTS

1 tablespoon apple cider vinegar
1 cup chopped honeydew melon
1 medium kiwi, peeled
½ cup hulled strawberries
½ cup plain kombucha
1½ cups sparkling water

---

1 In a large blender, combine the vinegar, melon, kiwi, strawberries, and kombucha.

2 Blend the ingredients on high until thoroughly combined and frothy.

3 Add the water gradually and continue blending until desired consistency is reached.

4 Consume immediately or store tightly sealed and unrefrigerated up to 4 hours.

KEY INGREDIENT: Kombucha

The fermentation process used to create kombucha generates a plentiful amount of healthy bacteria known as probiotics. These probiotics line your digestive tract, assist with absorption of nutrients, and help fight off infection and illness. And further, probiotics help to stabilize the pH of the vagina so that healthy bacteria can thrive, thereby helping women avoid bacterial infections such as yeast infections. The probiotics will also help boost your gut flora, which will in turn support your immune system. Kombucha is able to support the body's overall health and well-being naturally, but because some people find the flavor undesirable, it is recommended that you combine it with delicious additions like the ones found in this recipe. Maximizing kombucha's benefits, apple cider vinegar contains enzymes that effectively combat inflammation and irritation in the gut. By joining kombucha, ACV, and vibrant foods in this healthy drink, any woman can support her immune system with ample amounts of nutrients, phytochemicals, and antioxidants.

Per Serving

Calories: 70 | Fat: 0.5 g | Protein: 1 g | Sodium: 45 mg
Fiber: 3 g | Carbohydrates: 18 g | Sugar: 13 g

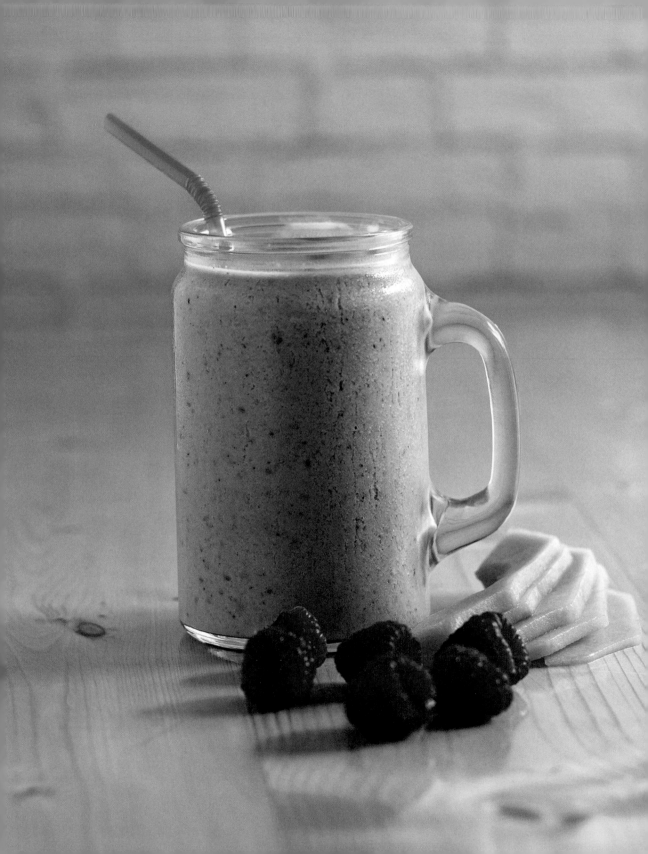

CREAMY CANTALOUPE-BERRY WITH FIGS AND FIZZ

Serves 2

INGREDIENTS

1 tablespoon apple cider vinegar
½ cup chopped cantaloupe
½ cup raspberries
1 medium fig
1½ cups low-fat plain Greek yogurt
1 cup ice
½ cup plain kombucha
1½ cups seltzer water

1 In a large blender, combine the vinegar, cantaloupe, raspberries, fig, yogurt, ice, and kombucha.

2 Blend the ingredients on high until thoroughly combined and frothy.

3 Add seltzer water gradually and continue blending until desired consistency is reached.

4 Consume immediately or store tightly sealed and refrigerated up to 4 hours. Shake well to revive fizz before serving.

KEY INGREDIENT: Raspberries

In the battle for breast, heart, and colon health, a clean diet of whole foods is highly recommended. Vibrant ingredients such as raspberries provide astounding amounts of nutrients in every serving. High in vitamin C and the mineral manganese, raspberries not only satisfy daily requirements for nutrients but also supply protective antioxidants that combat free radical damage that can lead to negative changes throughout the body. Degrading cell health adversely affects the tissues, organs, and systems, leading to dysfunctions that can wreak havoc on the body and brain over time. With delightful foods like raspberries combining with enzyme-rich apple cider vinegar in this recipe, prevention never tasted so sweet!

Per Serving
Calories: 180 | Fat: 4 g | Protein: 18 g | Sodium: 70 mg
Fiber: 3 g | Carbohydrates: 20 g | Sugar: 15 g

TWO-TONE PIE IN A GLASS

Serves 2

INGREDIENTS

1 tablespoon apple cider vinegar
1 cup blueberries
1 medium peach, pitted
½ cup low-fat granola
1 teaspoon ground cinnamon
¼ teaspoon ground cloves
2 cups low-fat vanilla Greek yogurt

1   Combine all the ingredients in a large blender.

2   Blend the ingredients on high until thoroughly combined and frothy.

3   Consume immediately or store tightly sealed and refrigerated up to 4 hours.

KEY INGREDIENT: Oats

Heart disease is the number one health risk for American women, yet not enough women make heart health a top priority. Luckily oats are an easy way to take care of heart health. The soluble fiber in oats can help reduce blood cholesterol, which may reduce the risk for heart disease. With plentiful benefits that range from colon cleansing and fighting inflammation to reducing the amount of "bad" cholesterol in the blood, the fiber in oats is an essential addition to any woman's diet. Ridding the colon of unhealthy bits of undigested debris, maximizing nutrient absorption, and increasing the amount of natural flora in the gut, the gel-like substance created by fiber (like that found in oats) can help improve digestion, immunity, and even cognitive processes that can be interrupted by digestion-related issues and complications. When you include oats in apple cider vinegar drinks, the benefits become even greater. Oats' naturally occurring nutrients become heightened with the protective enzymes of ACV that scour the body for toxins, inflammatory proteins, and free radicals naturally and deliciously!

Per Serving
Calories: 440 | Fat: 14 g | Protein: 25 g | Sodium: 100 mg
Fiber: 6 g | Carbohydrates: 57 g | Sugar: 41 g

SWEET BEETS AND GREENS WITH SPICE

Serves 2

INGREDIENTS

1 tablespoon apple cider vinegar
1 medium red beet, roasted and peeled
1 medium yellow beet, roasted and peeled
1 cup spinach leaves
1 teaspoon peeled and grated fresh gingerroot
1 teaspoon honey
2 cups purified water (pH-balanced)

1 In a large blender, combine the vinegar, beets, spinach, ginger, and honey.

2 Blend the ingredients on high until thoroughly combined and frothy.

3 Add the water gradually and continue blending until desired consistency is reached.

4 Consume immediately or store tightly sealed and unrefrigerated up to 4 hours.

KEY INGREDIENT: Beets

Beets contain an incredible amount of nutrition. While soothing the respiratory system, regulating hormones, providing the gut with healthy doses of fiber, and offering protective phytochemicals, beets prove to be powerhouses when it comes to women's health. The antioxidants in beets, called betalains, have several health benefits, including the ability to fight breast cancer cells, combat cell degradation, and safeguard the systems to which those cells belong. Beets also help reduce blood pressure and safeguard your heart health—an important issue for women. Because beets' sweet, earthy flavor complements apple cider vinegar's tartness so well, it's no surprise that these two ingredients also complement one another's nutritional content. Adding essential vitamins, minerals, and phytochemicals to ACV's rich enzyme stores, beets are able to satisfy the body's nutritional needs while also promoting the health of the immune system, reproductive system, and even vision. Any woman in search of a drink to better her health need search no further than this delightful recipe!

Per Serving
Calories: 42 | Fat: 0 g | Protein: 2 g | Sodium: 60 mg
Fiber: 2 g | Carbohydrates: 10 g | Sugar: 7 g

VERY BERRY MEDLEY WITH CREAM

Serves 2

INGREDIENTS

1 tablespoon apple cider vinegar
½ cup hulled strawberries
½ cup blueberries
½ cup raspberries
1½ cups low-fat plain Greek yogurt
½ cup plain kombucha
1 cup ice

1 Combine all the ingredients in a large blender.

2 Blend the ingredients on high until thoroughly combined and frothy.

3 Consume immediately or store tightly sealed and refrigerated up to 4 hours.

KEY INGREDIENT: Greek Yogurt

The inclusion of Greek yogurt in the daily diet is especially important for women due to its plentiful calcium and protein. Bone diseases like osteoporosis affect women more than men, making calcium intake a priority, especially for older women. Because it is made from a highly concentrated form of milk, you actually get more calcium from Greek yogurt than you do from a glass of milk. Meanwhile, protein is needed for everything from muscle development to the health of the skin, hair, and nails, making this drink a dream for all women. Greek yogurt is also packed with probiotics that can help boost the immune system and decrease stomach issues. Adding apple cider vinegar to a Greek yogurt–infused drink like this one serves to better women's health with each creamy sip.

Per Serving
Calories: 220 | Fat: 5 g | Protein: 23 g | Sodium: 85 mg
Fiber: 4 g | Carbohydrates: 22 g | Sugar: 15 g

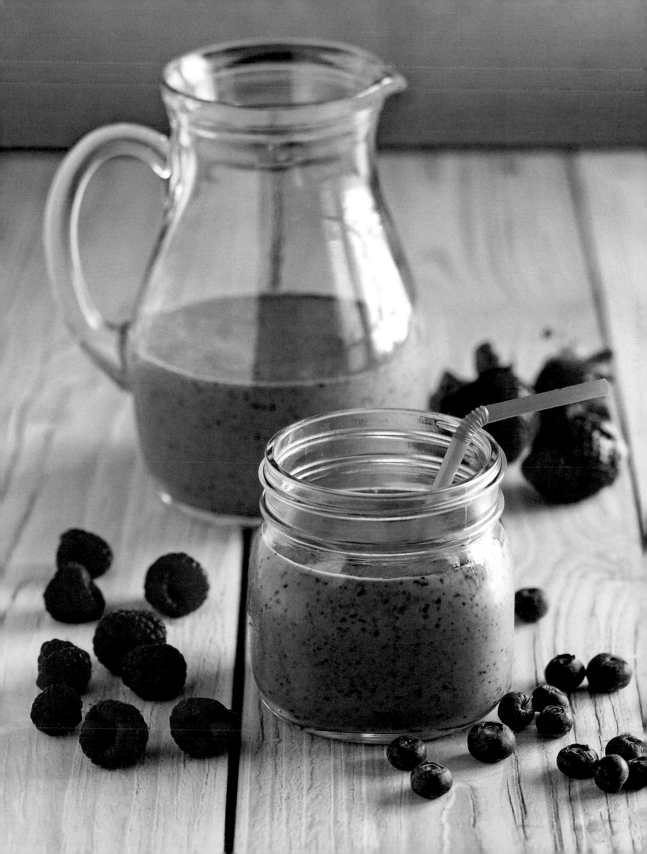

NUTS GALORE!

Serves 2

INGREDIENTS

1 tablespoon apple cider vinegar
½ cup whole, shelled cashews
½ cup whole, shelled walnuts
1 tablespoon ground flaxseed
2 tablespoons honey
1 cup ice
1 cup unsweetened vanilla almond
  milk
1 cup low-fat plain Greek yogurt

---

1 Combine all the ingredients in
   a large blender.

2 Blend the ingredients on high
   until thoroughly combined and
   frothy.

3 Consume immediately or store
   tightly sealed and refrigerated
   up to 4 hours.

KEY INGREDIENT: Flaxseeds

Packed with healthy omega-3 fatty acids, flaxseeds add countless health benefits and a nutty richness to this recipe. In addition to producing healthy, protein-rich hair, glowing skin, and strong nails, flaxseeds also provide women with benefits that directly promote healthy cell growth and maintenance in the breasts, brain, blood, and cervix. Assisting in the absorption of nutrients, flaxseeds support the health of bones throughout the body that could otherwise succumb to osteoporosis or osteoarthritis. In addition, the high levels of omega-3 fatty acids in flaxseeds help prevent the hardening of arteries and keep plaque from being deposited in the arteries, helping the cardiovascular system. The addition of apple cider vinegar brings enzymes that cleanse the body of toxins and harmful free radicals that could potentially cause illness. By combining these two ingredients with other clean, whole foods, any woman desiring to look and feel her best while aiming for total wellness can sip her way there with this delicious recipe.

Per Serving
Calories: 690 | Fat: 49 g | Protein: 26 g | Sodium: 140 mg
Fiber: 5 g | Carbohydrates: 46 g | Sugar: 25 g

CREAMY VANILLA SWEET POTATO PIE

Serves 2

INGREDIENTS

1 tablespoon apple cider vinegar
1 large sweet potato, baked and peeled
1 teaspoon ground cinnamon
¼ teaspoon ground cloves
1 cup ice
1 cup nonfat plain Greek yogurt
1 cup purified water (pH-balanced)

1 In a large blender, combine the vinegar, sweet potato, cinnamon, cloves, ice, and yogurt.

2 Blend the ingredients on high until thoroughly combined and frothy.

3 Add the water gradually and continue blending until desired consistency is reached.

4 Consume immediately or store tightly sealed and refrigerated up to 4 hours.

KEY INGREDIENT: Sweet Potato

Sweet potatoes have long been known as rich sources of vitamin A and lycopene, but they also contain vitamin B_6, vitamin C, and minerals such as manganese and potassium. Because sweet potatoes are a slow-releasing carbohydrate, they will not spike your blood sugar levels and will leave you feeling fuller longer, so you will have balanced energy and be less likely to snack on unhealthy foods. As an added benefit, the vitamin A in sweet potatoes protects the health and well-being of the eyes, ensuring that debilitating diseases such as glaucoma are kept at bay. With apple cider vinegar drinks like this one, a woman in search of an all-natural approach to health can find energizing nutrients that support the functioning of all of the body's systems. With sweetness from the potatoes, richness from the calcium-packed Greek yogurt, and potent enzymes that flourish in every ounce of ACV, this drink recipe makes a delicious and nutritious addition to any woman's diet.

Per Serving
Calories: 150 | Fat: 0.5 g | Protein: 13 g | Sodium: 75 mg
Fiber: 4 g | Carbohydrates: 24 g | Sugar: 10 g

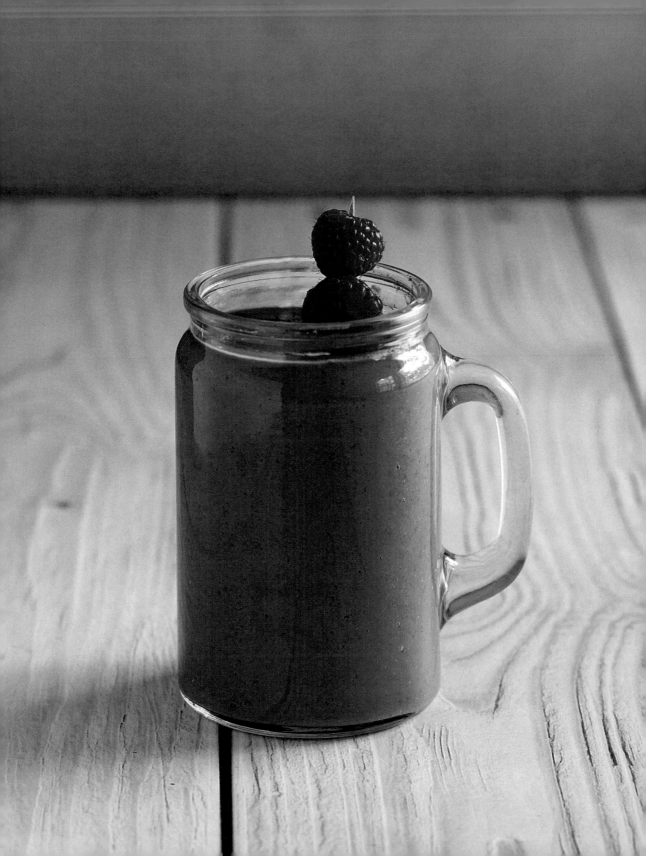

RASPBERRY CREAM WITH GINGER AND SPICE

Serves 2

INGREDIENTS

1 tablespoon apple cider vinegar

2 cups raspberries

1 teaspoon peeled and grated fresh gingerroot

1/4 teaspoon ground cloves

1 cup low-fat plain Greek yogurt

1 cup ice

1 cup purified water (pH-balanced)

1 In a large blender, combine the vinegar, raspberries, ginger, cloves, yogurt, and ice.

2 Blend the ingredients on high until thoroughly combined and frothy.

3 Add the water gradually and continue blending until desired consistency is reached.

4 Consume immediately or store tightly sealed and refrigerated up to 4 hours.

KEY INGREDIENT: Ginger

With potent compounds called gingerols, ginger adds a sweet spiciness to any apple cider vinegar drink and also packs in the nutrition. Gingerols not only fight inflammation and free radical damage, but they also make your skin glow by soothing out red, irritated skin and by protecting your collagen stores, which help your skin look younger. Helping to alleviate respiratory distress and stomach discomfort, ginger has long been used throughout the world to naturally restore the body's cells, organs, and systems to a healthy balance. In addition, it also helps prevent cardiovascular disease, boosts circulation, and increases libido. When combined with antioxidant-rich berries and spices, along with protein- and calcium-rich yogurt, the ginger in this ACV drink is even more potent for overall health and well-being. Any woman in search of the perfect protein-rich breakfast, satisfying snack, or delectable dessert can turn to this quick and easy recipe that's as effective at protecting and promoting health as it is delicious!

Per Serving

Calories: 150 | Fat: 3 g | Protein: 13 g | Sodium: 45 mg
Fiber: 8 g | Carbohydrates: 20 g | Sugar: 10 g

US/Metric Conversion Chart

VOLUME CONVERSIONS

US Volume Measure	Metric Equivalent
⅛ teaspoon	0.5 milliliter
¼ teaspoon	1 milliliter
½ teaspoon	2 milliliters
1 teaspoon	5 milliliters
½ tablespoon	7 milliliters
1 tablespoon (3 teaspoons)	15 milliliters
2 tablespoons (1 fluid ounce)	30 milliliters
¼ cup (4 tablespoons)	60 milliliters
⅓ cup	90 milliliters
½ cup (4 fluid ounces)	125 milliliters
⅔ cup	160 milliliters
¾ cup (6 fluid ounces)	180 milliliters
1 cup (16 tablespoons)	250 milliliters
1 pint (2 cups)	500 milliliters
1 quart (4 cups)	1 liter (about)

WEIGHT CONVERSIONS

US Weight Measure	Metric Equivalent
½ ounce	15 grams
1 ounce	30 grams
2 ounces	60 grams
3 ounces	85 grams
¼ pound (4 ounces)	115 grams
½ pound (8 ounces)	225 grams
¾ pound (12 ounces)	340 grams
1 pound (16 ounces)	454 grams

OVEN TEMPERATURE CONVERSIONS

Degrees Fahrenheit	Degrees Celsius
200 degrees F	95 degrees C
250 degrees F	120 degrees C
275 degrees F	135 degrees C
300 degrees F	150 degrees C
325 degrees F	160 degrees C
350 degrees F	180 degrees C
375 degrees F	190 degrees C
400 degrees F	205 degrees C
425 degrees F	220 degrees C
450 degrees F	230 degrees C

BAKING PAN SIZES

American	Metric
8 x 1½ inch round baking pan	20 x 4 cm cake tin
9 x 1½ inch round baking pan	23 x 3.5 cm cake tin
11 x 7 x 1½ inch baking pan	28 x 18 x 4 cm baking tin
13 x 9 x 2 inch baking pan	30 x 20 x 5 cm baking tin
2 quart rectangular baking dish	30 x 20 x 3 cm baking tin
15 x 10 x 2 inch baking pan	30 x 25 x 2 cm baking tin (Swiss roll tin)
9 inch pie plate	22 x 4 or 23 x 4 cm pie plate
7 or 8 inch springform pan	18 or 20 cm springform or loose bottom cake tin
9 x 5 x 3 inch loaf pan	23 x 13 x 7 cm or 2 lb narrow loaf or pate tin
1½ quart casserole	1.5 liter casserole
2 quart casserole	2 liter casserole

Index